The events described in *Through The Fire* are similar to what Job in the Bible experienced.

- Pete Dechat is a 21st Century Job.
- People tell him how lucky he is to be alive.
- He knows different.
- "God brought me through the fire."
- Pete will tell you things as he learned about them.

Mostly after awakening from five months in a coma.

Through The Fire

The True Story of a 21st Century Job

Pete Dechat

Copyright 2018 by Pete Dechat
Cover design by Marti Dobkins
Published by UCS PRESS
ISBN: 978-0-943247-10-6

Most of the Bible verses quoted in this book are from the New King James Version (NKJV) translation.

NOTE: Some names in this book have been changed for reasons of privacy.

Contact the publisher via publisher@ucspress.com for discount pricing for large quantity orders.
First printing April 2018.

View the author's testimony at

https://www.youtube.com/watch?v=4Cgv6ASLFK0&feature=youtu.be

About the Author

This is Pete Dechat's first book. A labor of love by a man who went from wanting to be a rock star to telling everyone he can about the Creator of the stars in the heavens.

He literally went Through The Fire. His ministry is sharing with people in the United States and other countries how God brought him through that fire.

The son of Andrew Frank Dechat and Monika Lore Dechat, was born in 1971 at George Washington University Hospital in Washington, D.C.

He graduated from Osborne Park High School in Manassas, Virginia.

Pete lives with his wife Judy and daughter Rebekah on Virginia land that includes goats, chickens, gardens and fruit trees.

In Loving Memory

Gabriella Louise Dechat

"Gabi"

November 2, 2002 – July 10, 2007

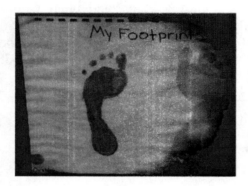

This is Gabi's footprint found on a partially-burned sheet of paper after the fire. It is a reminder that she left her footprint on the hearts of all those who loved her.

Dedication

To Mom and Dad. They were there
for me when I needed them the most – after
God brought me through the fire.

Introduction

My story is like a diamond. There are many facets, and each brings about another level of beauty to the overall story. It's too hard for me to choose a singular focal point because there are too many things worthy of sharing.

However, once you've read this true story, you will have no doubt about what the ultimate focus is in my life.

This story will speak to anyone who has gone through a hard time, a struggle, crisis or pain – really anyone over the age of five probably fits that description.

I see things and tell things from a Christian perspective. Even if you're not a Christian, I pray that if you have gone through what seems to be too much for you, or you know someone who's struggling, my story will be of special encouragement. The majority of people I've told my story to have found it inspiring, and some even life-changing.

It is common for people to let circumstances define them, and they live as a victim. It is true that we can be a victim of something negative happening in our lives, but choosing to live as a victim is just that – a choice. "Woe is me" can easily become a way of life. It can consume you. To me, that's like looking at the ground instead of at the sky. You need to change your perspective, or change what you focus on. The roses. The trees. The lakes. The mountains. There are too many beautiful things in this life to only see the negative. Feeling sorry for yourself is seeing the glass half-empty instead of half-full. That's like being half-alive, which is also half-dead. You are robbing yourself of the fullness life has to offer. I know from experiencing tragedy but more importantly from experiencing victories.

My circumstances don't define me. The One living in me does. Jesus said in John 10:10, "The thief does not come except to steal, and to kill, and to destroy. I have come that they may have life, and that they may have it more abundantly." But neither Jesus nor the *thief* can do it unless YOU allow them to.

Someone recently asked me how I was able to avoid having pity parties because of getting burned on 96% of my body, and the many months of surgeries and rehab. I told him, "Not living like a victim is my choice. Sure, I could let myself moan and groan like I was a victim, and many would believe I had the right to behave that way. But bad things happen to good people all the time. So my attitude was 'Why NOT me?'"

Why has God blessed me with all He has? I don't know. I know that when you are faithful with little He has a way of promoting you to bigger things. But it doesn't mean bad things won't keep coming your way. I don't even know myself well enough to understand the trust He has put in me to share this story. But I am thankful He is allowing me to serve Him in this way.

To God be the glory!

Pete Dechat

Who would want to bomb Mickey?

Something caused the walls of our two-story home in the Orlando, Florida suburb of Sanford to shake. Seconds later there was a loud explosion.

I thought a nuclear bomb had gone off. *Disney World was the only thing close, but who would want to bomb Mickey?*

My four-year-old daughter Gabriella – Gabi was sleeping in our bedroom, which was on the first floor. My stepson Jimmy, who was 10, was in his upstairs bedroom. My wife Gladys and I were in the office where I ran my company out of, Professional Window Treatments of Central Florida, which was also on the second floor.

I was still in my underwear, and had an untouched cup of coffee on my desk. I was talking on the phone to a neighbor who installed blinds and shutters for me. My wife was behind me, faxing in an order when the explosion happened.

We ran out of the office. At this point I had no idea that our house was even on fire. I just knew we had to get out of there. Gladys went down the stairs as fast as she could. She went through the living room and out the front door. When I ran out of the office, I started toward Jimmy's room first, but I saw Jimmy already coming down the hallway. So I headed down the steps as well.

When I got to the open front door, I stopped – one hand on either side of the door frame, realizing Gabi wouldn't know what to do. I turned back and ran for her.

Gabi

I had no thoughts of what could happen when I went to find Gabi – just that I had to get her out. It didn't matter what would happen to me as long as I could save my baby. I didn't consider the danger I was putting myself in. I just instinctively ran to find her. I was absolutely certain I was going to get her out. Failing was not an option.

In my haste I ran upstairs to her room, forgetting she was downstairs in our bed. I was so upset I wasted those valuable seconds. When I finally got back down to the master bedroom and opened the door, smoke billowed out. The fire was deafening. I had no idea how loud fire could actually be. Smoke was getting into my lungs. The sound of the flames was like a steady roar. The smoke was so thick I couldn't even see my hand in front of my face.

I stumbled across the debris making my way to the bed. I kept yelling as loud as I could. "Gabi, Gabi! Daddy's here to save you! Where are you?" She didn't respond. All I could hear were Gabi's cries, but I couldn't tell where they were coming from.

As a parent, you understand the different cries of your child. You can tell when she's hurt, when she's tired, or when she's just cranky. This was like none of those. These cries were different. They sounded like the cries of someone who had lost hope.

I finally made it to the bed. It was covered with tattered drywall and broken 2x4's. With one hand I lifted the debris, desperately searching with the other to find my little girl. All the time continuing to call out for her, and hearing nothing in response but those haunting cries. I can still hear those cries today.

The fire was getting closer. I was standing right in front of the open closet door with my back to it. This closet was about 12 feet deep. I wanted to see how close the flames were so I turned. What I saw could be anyone's rendition of what hell might look like. Inferno would be understating it. I had never seen fire so intense. It was 10 to12 feet away from me, floor to ceiling.

The intensity of my search ramped up to match the danger I now realized I was in. At this point, I didn't even feel the heat. I didn't feel any pain. I didn't even realize the struggle I was having to breathe. Finally overcome by the smoke, I blacked out. My body slumped onto the bed while the flames got closer.

It must have been an angel that woke me, shouting, "Get out now!" My back had been facing the fire in the master bedroom, but from the time I heard this voice, to when I stumbled out of the house and off the front porch, seemed like only a few seconds. The first person I saw was Jimmy. He looked blistered and was standing in a way that looked like he was in a great deal of pain.

My competitive nature bloomed early

Early on, I was competitive in the classroom, and in sports.

I vividly remember being in a spelling bee in the second grade. It got down to the last two of us. I went first. My word (in second grade, mind you) orangutan – even though the teacher pronounced it "orangutang." I spelled it out exactly as it sounded, which obviously was wrong.

My opponent was given the word *brown*. That might have been the first time in my life I mumbled to myself, *You kidding me?* To this day that still bothers me. The girl was practically grinning when she spelled *b r o w n.*

At that same school, there was a teacher that would kick one of those rubber *kick balls* way above the school, and I was able to catch it.

Now to be fair, perspective for a first or second grader is not exactly to scale. But he wasn't pooch punting it. He was giving it his all. And those balls fly when you kick them. My arms stung and would turn bright red, but I would do it over and over again. I guess since none of the other kids could catch it, they wouldn't stick around. I learned a lesson that has stuck with me all these years:

Whatever you do, give it your best effort. And don't give up.

Latchkey kids

Marion Dechat (now Fera) is my older sister by two-and-one-half years. As latchkey children, we basically raised ourselves. Our parents were never home. They worked in Washington, D.C. They left before we woke up, and didn't get home until 6-7 p.m.

We had to wake ourselves, dress ourselves, and feed ourselves. It was great for me because this level of responsibility as a child served me well as an adult. I sometimes wonder how kids today would survive that.

Our family did not do a lot of things together, but I wasn't unhappy as a child. I was very good at entertaining myself. My dad also did a good job showing me how much *fun* splitting wood, and other chores could be just like in Tom Sawyer. My parents' focus was on their jobs – both worked for the government. It's funny how subconsciously we really do admire our parents. When all the other kids were saying they wanted to grow up to be policemen, firemen, athletes, or astronauts, I had the exotic aspiration of growing up to work for the government – just like Mom and Dad.

There was no evidence of religion in our home – not even grace said before meals. We went to church only at Christmas and Easter. Going to church was just what you had to endure to get to the sweets or treats when we got home.

My sister and I ended up in different high schools because of rezoning. She stayed at Garfield High School and I went to Osborne Park High School.

I have to mention this: when I was younger, it was never a problem with my friends coming over and my sister being there. What got weird was when we got older and my friends started noticing my sister. It's never cool to hear from your friends how hot they think your sister is. Awkward.

My parents would not let me participate in organized team sports. I don't know if it was because of the cost, the time, or both. At 16, I started working out every day. I only weighed 120 pounds, but I could do 50 pull-ups, 100 push-ups, and 100 sit-ups all in five minutes.

My mom didn't like that I was working out because she thought I wanted to fight. I explained, "It's not because I want to fight, it's because I want people to think twice before picking a fight with me."

Building Fort Apache

In the eighth or ninth grade some buddies and I decided to build our own private hangout. We called it Fort Apache. A three-room structure that was suspended totally off the ground, positioned against several trees that provided strong, stable support. The rooms were connected by doorways, and each room was at a different level above the ground; maybe about 800 total square feet of indoor space. Because of the trees, each room had a unique shape.

It was a mile back in the woods behind our community. We kept it our secret.

As the derelicts we were, my friends and I would diligently sneak out almost every night, steal lumber from a nearby construction site, and somehow carry it through the woods in the dark.

I'm pretty sure our craftsmanship wouldn't meet any building code, but it was quite the feat for us. We even tar-papered the roof.

One of the funniest memories I have was a warm summer evening. A bunch of us were heading to the fort at dusk.

We decided to race. I got way ahead of everyone so I stopped to see how far behind they were. It was pretty dark, but I could hear their voices and could tell they weren't far behind. When I turned back to start running to the fort, one inch from my face, was the biggest, ugliest spider I'd ever seen. It was on a huge spider web spanning about six feet in diameter. It was a bluish-grey color and had a one-and-one-half-inch fat body.

My breathing moved the web back and forth letting it sway perilously close to my face. I screamed like a little girl.

When they asked what was wrong, I almost couldn't get the word out. I stuttered out *sp-p-p-spider*. They all laughed at me.

As far as I know, Mom and Dad never knew I was sneaking out at nights. From their always-long workdays, getting up and leaving so early in the morning, and getting back home so late in the evening, they probably treasured their sleeping hours.

Self-taught strummer

I started playing bass guitar only because my friend Chad got a guitar about six months earlier for Christmas. He had been taking lessons and he told me, "Get a bass guitar and we can start a band."

I bought an old Univox bass and a small 30w Gorilla bass amp. I'd never played bass, or any other instrument for that matter. As soon as I got it home, I plugged it in and popped in my Billy Idol cassette tape. The song that came on was *Mony Mony*. I didn't even know how to tune the bass, or that it needed to be tuned, but was able to figure out how to play along with the song anyway.

When Chad came over so I could show him, he only said one word, "Jerk!" He said it with love I'm sure.

We named our *band* Apache after our childhood tree house. It was only the two of us in it. Our primary audience and most fervent fans, also the two of us. We did jam for a few friends. But mostly just dreamed.

The windshield battered my face

When I was 15 my front teeth were knocked out in a horrible car accident. The hole in my chin needed 72 stitches. I blew blood bubbles out of the hole. It was big enough to stick my pinky finger through.

My jaw was dislocated and broken in three places. The front part was not just broken but shattered to where it couldn't be rebuilt, so there is a part under the upper front bridge where the bone is missing. No one can see it except the dentists when they work on my teeth.

There were four of us in the car. The driver was a young lady, Trish. She was big into the punk movement, as was my friend Ron in the front passenger seat.

I sat in the back behind Trish. Chad sat beside me right behind Ron. We were not into the punk movement, but at that time we had friends that represented every facet of society.

Trish drove with her left foot on the brakes and right foot on the gas. Bad idea. They were building out Potomac Mills Mall, and there were many new roads and stoplights.

I had fallen asleep in the backseat, so I didn't witness how the accident happened. I was told that we were coming up to one of the new lights when a huge station wagon stopped in front of us. Trish panicked and mistakenly slammed down on the gas instead of the brakes. So she sped up instead of slowing down, slamming into the station wagon at top speed.

None of us wore our seat belts, so I flew over the driver's seat and smashed into the windshield face first.

I remember Trish saying she thought she lost her eye, but it was her eyelid that was ripped off. She also had a broken arm,

Ron was the worst off. He had a fractured skull and his nose was peeled back.

Chad had the best luck that day. He just sprained his knee.

He still laughs that I kept coming to him every couple of minutes asking, "Hey Chad, Is it bad?"

"Yes, it's bad, Pete."

"Hey, Chad, Is it bad?"

"Yes, it's really bad."

"Hey, Chad, Is it bad?"

"No, it's actually ok."

I kept repeating things because I had a concussion.

Chad later told me, "You kept asking me that, and alternating blowing bubbles out of the hole in your chin. I swear you were smiling."

My dentist was the most upset of everyone because I was the only one in our family that had perfect teeth. I had to wear *flappers* until they made my permanent bridges. They are expensive, about $10,000, and the top one has to be replaced every ten years or so. The bottom is still the original one, over thirty years old now.

Through the course of the next year after the car crash, bone fragments kept making their way out through the roof of my mouth as the front part of my upper jaw was shattered so badly.

Me, a punching bag

My parents went out of town that weekend, but since I had to work I stayed behind.

The boys I hung around with most that particular year were brothers, Tommy and Sonny. Their grandparents owned a music shop. Their dad was both a crack and heroin addict at the same time – and functioning. His addiction was so bad that he ended up having half his hand amputated because of the heroin abuse.

Tommy got into the same drugs as his dad, but Sonny, who was a few years younger, only drank and smoked pot. The three of us went out to a party. I didn't really know anyone there, but I was social so I fit in.

Out of nowhere I got blindsided with a punch to the side of my head. The guy was a 250-pound football player. He caught me totally off guard. Before I knew it, one guy pulled the bandana from my head to around my neck and held me in place from behind, while several other guys pounded on me. Any time I moved forward, he pulled me back like a dog on a choke collar.

I was only able to look up once and I made it count. I knocked the guy down that was in front of me. Other than that I felt like the side of beef in the Rocky movie. They eventually wore themselves out and stopped.

My false teeth were knocked out. I was looking around for them when this skinny punk came up to me. He yelled, "You hit me!" He started a new round in the fight.

He was right, I did hit him. He was the guy I knocked down. The rest of the team formed a circle around us to see how he'd do on his own. He was probably three or four inches taller, and about twenty pounds heavier, but I took him down and was beating the snot out of him – remember, I may have been light, but it was all in my biceps. I could do fifty pull-ups easily.

When they saw him losing they all jumped in on me. I got the guy in a choke hold and told him, "They might kill me tonight, but I'm taking you with me."

I really thought that was going to be the outcome; that they were going to beat me to death. I remember letting go and hitting the closest guy to me. Unfortunately, he was the only one trying to pull people off of me. Yikes, he jumped in too. In a moment of desperation I cried out, "You're killing me! You're killing me!"

With that they finally stopped.

I looked like the elephant man, totally disfigured.

I got helped to my car where I found my two *loyal* friends, Tommy and Sonny, cowering. It turns out that Tommy had started the fight. They beat me up because they knew I was with him.

When we got back to their house, their dad looked at me, then looked at them and said in disgust, "There is no excuse for why you two don't look like him," and walked away.

Rock star

In no way was I a positive role model during my teen years. Knucklehead is a word that sums up those years best. I did a lot of things I should not have done. That behavior was really on display when I was bass guitarist with the thrash metal band, Calibra.

It was maybe a few months after the beating that a drummer who knew of me, asked me to audition for Calibra. I was really surprised I made it. That group was so talented. I was good, but I can honestly say that I was the weak link. At that time I'd never taken a lesson, but was able to pick things up by ear quickly.

I felt like I needed to learn more and started taking lessons. I wanted to catch up to the level of talent in the rest of the group. The instructor was brilliant, and extremely talented. He was playing for the band Foghat at the time. As talented as he was, I stopped taking lessons because he was trying to teach me techniques that didn't seem relevant in my view with what we played.

(Later, because of my friends Tim, who played drums, and Fernando, I joined them in a jazz band.)

Calibra was a wild and crazy time for me. Sex, drugs, and rock and roll was not a saying for me – it was a lifestyle. I was one of those guys who'd take his shirt off and jam like crazy, jumping out into the crowd. Someone recently found a picture online from one of our shows. Ahh, the things that come back to haunt you.

Then I saw the writing on the wall. I saw many extremely talented, yet starving musicians. At the time I was a janitor by day, and they needed ME to buy them something to eat?! It didn't look like the road I wanted to be on.

The road to superstar salesman

I started my working life at a Giant Food supermarket at 16. I bagged and loaded groceries for customers, and then moved into a porter (janitor) position. I was such a bonehead that I was offered the option to quit or be fired after it was found out that another knucklehead and I had stolen a keg of beer. I chose the former.

I then worked at McDonald's in the grill area. I was actually accepted by two companies, the other being Chili's, which would've actually paid $1 per hour more. I took the job at McDonald's because another friend of mine – Fernando – got hired the same day I did.

After the first day he quit. I learned that I should never base my decisions on what a friend is going to do. I eventually got promoted to janitor, which I did full time while playing in the band. After determining I wasn't going to be a rock star, I asked my manager one Friday after my shift what he thought about me quitting the band and going into management. He said, "Cut your hair and start Monday." I moved to different locations in northern Virginia.

I was eventually very heavily recruited by Schwan's frozen food. I was finally convinced to take the job, and worked as a sales person. I flourished there and quickly was top salesman in my region, and went on to be the number two sales rep in the entire company (that's pretty good considering there were over 8,000 sales people nationwide). I was promoted to sales manager in Manassas, and worked there for nearly seven years in that position.

They decided to redistrict, and a divisional manager that had cursed me out early in my managerial career was taking over my facility. When asked what I thought about going to work for him, I said, "I won't. I'll transfer, or leave the company."

That's how I ended up in Florida. A division manager that knew of me had an opening and took me.

John Nootenboom was the person who originally talked to me about joining Schwan's. He was a sales rep at the time. He also was promoted, and worked as a sales manager at the Manassas location while I was there. We both were highly successful. He ended up leaving the company before I did, and he started Professional Window Treatments. He had been begging me to leave Schwan's to come work for him, but there was no way he could compensate me enough to do it.

But when my wife and I saw all the new houses going up near where we lived, we asked about buying a franchise from him. We took the profit from the sale of our home in Manassas, and bought a house to live in – that would later become a rental property – put a contract on another house (the one where the angel saved my life), and bought Professional Window Treatments of Central Florida.

There was a corporate decision to downsize at Schwan's, so they had to let either myself, or the other manager working in my office go. I should have let the other manager keep his job and worked the blind business full time. But I was scared, and didn't really know enough about it at the time. They chose to keep me and I accepted. The employees there didn't like it. It was not an easy situation for anyone there.

They allowed me to promote some assistants. One salesman that had transferred from another region and was highly successful, wanted that job badly; but I didn't think he was a natural leader. When he asked for examples of who I thought was a good leader, I named several, including Washington and Grant.

I made the mistake of saying even evil people could be considered great leaders – not because they were good people, but because they got people to follow them. I said, "Even Hitler could be considered a great leader because he got an entire nation to do the unthinkable."

From that, it was twisted into "Pete thinks Hitler is great."

Flatly opposite from what I actually think. Any remaining loyalty withered away. I decided at that point it was best to part ways, and start working full time for our blind company. In the first three months, I produced as much profit as I'd have earned in an entire year at Schwan's. I actually worked less at that point than any other point in my adult life.

I marketed by mailing flyers to houses that were newly constructed, and knocked on doors whenever I saw people home.

I was the primary sales force, installer, marketer, and accountant – chief cook and bottle washer in a manner of speaking – of my business. I had two people who helped as contractors. My neighbor was the main one. He lived right next door, and did much of the installations. He was the one I was on the phone with when I thought Disney World might have been nuked.

I had married Gladys in September 2001. She was my second wife. My first wife was a good friend of mine. But I was a horrible husband to her. I was married more to my work than to her. Not that she didn't have her own faults. I just know that I was the reason it didn't work out. We amicably split, and I know she's remarried. I hope he is better to her than I was. Everyone deserves that.

Daffy Duck

I loved my stepson Jimmy like he was my own son. My daughter Gabi loved him, and looked up to him. I have this wonderful photo where she was caught wearing his hat. Her expression of being *busted* was priceless.

Jimmy was protective of Gabi. One time she sat on a fire ant hill. Jimmy saw it, grabbed her off of it and stripped her clothes off to keep her from getting more bites. Very quick thinking on his part.

One of my favorite memories with him was when he was three or four. He went to a daycare close to our house in Manassas. I would go to pick him up early when they were all on the playground outside. I would let the kids chase me around all the while laughing like Daffy Duck. Just picture a mob of twenty or so toddlers trying to catch me.

I'm sure that could've been a huge liability for the daycare, but the teachers loved it when I came. It was a break for them because ALL the kids wanted to chase me.

Severed finger is no excuse

I loved softball. Really, I loved anything competitive. I was strong, and fast. I would be the guy that could cover the ENTIRE centerfield. I could also hit the ball far, but it was base-running speed that made me dangerous. I could get to third where most guys might only get to first or maybe second.

In Virginia I collected league championship shirts on several very competitive teams. I also played in Florida, but not long enough to reach any level of success with that team.

I was working at a customer's house while she was having her wooden floors replaced. Because of this, she had all the back doors open. As I ran out the front door to grab some more samples, the wind blew the door shut. The middle finger on my left hand got slammed in the door right where the lock plate was.

This literally cut through the bone right at the root of the fingernail. The skin on the underside of the finger was the only part still attached.

I calmly walked back into the kitchen, and said, "I think I need to go to the hospital."

I have never been faint at the sight of trauma, but when I looked at my finger move around freely in any direction – almost like a video game joystick – I felt my knees buckle.

The customer drove me to the hospital. For some reason, they insisted on an X-ray, even after I told them the bone was cut clear through. I sat waiting for the X-ray. And I sat, and I sat. Finally, after the fourth person had come, got X-rayed, and left, I spoke up. "I've been sitting for over an hour with my finger cut off. When is it my turn?"

I wasn't even on the list! They finally did the X-ray and confirmed what I had been telling them all along.

This male nurse came in.

"What do we do now?" I asked, "…tear it off like Ronnie Lott did?"

"Oh, not at all," he said.

I was surprised. "You've seen this before?"

His response makes me laugh even today. "No, but I read the manual."

We both laughed.

"Look here," he said, "this blood flow is coming from the tip of your finger back...this finger will be just fine."

By this time the numbing shot was wearing off. He proceeded to tear off the nail, and dig out the nail's root. Then he sewed the tip back on and wrapped me up.

One of my neighbors saw the injury and said, "That's got to be worth at least $50,000."

That's the problem with society today; people's first thought is lawsuit. No way would I sue. It wasn't the customer's fault I got my finger caught in her door. It was mine.

More painful than the injury was the $11,000 bill I got for getting the care I received. I have a picture of Gabi's fourth birthday where you can see my finger wrapped up.

Two weeks later I tapped on the tip of my finger. It didn't hurt. It was completely attached and healed.

After the original bill I got, I figured no thank you, I'll pull these stitches out myself, and I did. That night I played in a softball game. I was more worried about catching the ball awkward because the injury was on my glove hand.

Everything went fine.

Last birthday present from Gabi

The Rotavirus is a nasty intestinal illness that lasts three to ten days. Gabi was terribly sick. It started with throwing up, and transitioned to uncontrollable diarrhea. On my 36th birthday, she was very lethargic, so we dropped everything and took her to the hospital. They needed a stool sample from her, and she was so out of it that I needed to carry her. The bathroom was only fifteen feet away, but she let it all out before we were even half way there. I was covered in her poop.

"I've got your stool sample now."

The sample scraped off of me was positive for the disease. It would prove to be the last birthday present I would get from her. I scrubbed and scrubbed, but still got it. It started on a Monday. I was out of commission for seven days. I remember going to bed, still sick as a dog, Sunday night thinking *I need to work!*

I woke up Monday morning completely fine, as if it never happened.

John 3:16

My best friend, Tim Pemberton, gave me my first Bible as a Christmas present in 2003. I was 32. It made a wonderful coffee table ornament. I never even opened the book.

When I was setting up my window treatment business, I was shopping for a bank. While standing in line at Washington Mutual, a really nice black gentleman started talking to me. He said something to me that may as well have been Chinese.

When I asked for clarification, he said, "You don't go to church do you?"

"No."

He asked, "Do you have a Bible?"

"Yes."

"Go read John 3:16."

I'm a man of my word, so I did. But it didn't really mean anything to me.

A week or so later, I knocked on the door of people that just moved into their new house and didn't already have their windows covered with any sort of treatment. This couple, as it turned out, were pastors trying to revitalize a dying church. During my presentation, they invited me to the church. Very selfishly, I thought *if it helps me get this sale, I'll come to your church.*

I got the sale.

When I got home, I asked my wife what she thought about coming to church with me that Sunday. She agreed, and we went. It was an old building that had been added onto, and remodeled many times over its 100-plus years history, but it looked run-down and in desperate need of a little TLC.

The congregation was small, and very old. The average age seemed to be in the 70's, with several in their 90's. The church, once thriving, was now dying – quite literally.

I felt welcomed, and really enjoyed it. I got more involved, and within a few months I asked to be baptized. I became the treasurer, and ran the A/V system. My mom was actually offended that I wanted to be baptized.

"You were already baptized."

I contended that as an infant, it meant nothing to me. But now, this was an outward declaration of what was happening inside me.

The moment that I knew it was real – and I think anyone completely sold out to Jesus has that moment – was late one evening when I was driving home from a long day of working. A mile or so from home I pulled up to the train tracks as a train was passing. It was dark outside, and I had the Christian radio station playing. Having played music so many years, I always had the tendency to listen more to the music. Even though I could sing along with the words, they were really secondary to me. But that night I really zoomed in on the words:

". . . amazing love, how can it be . . . that you my King would die for me . . ."

That really hit me like a ton of bricks in the middle of my chest. Tears flowed uncontrollably. I was undone. *How is it that the king of the universe could sacrifice Himself for me?*

My relationship with Jesus, and my love for Him, for the first time was real in that moment.

Comatose

Five months of darkness

I did not know about anything that was going on around me or done to me all during the five months I was in a coma.

No out-of-body experience.

Nothing.

But I did have several reoccurring dreams that I remember very well. They seem very disjointed and unrelated, but in my mind I think it was my subconscious reliving the experience.

There was the dream that I was running into a burning house, where the walls were as paper. Sometimes I was looking for someone; sometimes I was just there. In that dream it was almost always dark outside.

Another dream I remember is that I was hung over a pit of fire – shackled in a way that my arms were outstretched and my legs so that they were together – the way Jesus was on the cross. Two evil beings were cutting the flesh off of my legs. Eventually that dream, which reoccurred frequently, came to a conclusion when I was helped down from where I was hung to be cared for. That dream never happened again from that point on.

In another dream I was on what seemed like a boat floating down a tropical river. But it was not really a boat. It was more like tree branches suspended quite high above the water. Each branch was long and about twelve inches in diameter. I couldn't see many other branches – only three or four – but they each had someone on them. I didn't communicate with anyone in any of those dreams.

One dream was me being in what seemed like a large sewage drain. It was dark, damp, and completely full of corpses and dismembered body parts. There was groaning, so I wasn't the only one alive in that dream. Everything was flowing very slowly, but I don't know to where. It gave me a feeling of it being inescapable.

The final dream I remember is one where I descended into a large glass jar, kind of shaped like the bottom three-fourths of an hour glass. Inside was like an entire world, and I was always searching for treasures. It was an epic dream that seemed to perpetuate and evolve as if it never ended. It was the dream that reoccurred the most, and I actually remember having a sense that I enjoyed that dream when it came.

No dream could have prepared me for the new realities that my life had become while I was asleep to the world.

There was no bomb

They induced my coma before the news spread around the country. Below is the headline that was posted on Tuesday July 10, 2007 at www.thenewyorktimes.com. And part of the news article:

Small Plane Crash in Florida Kills 5
By DENNIS BLANK and MARIA NEWMAN

SANFORD, Fla. July 10 — A small airplane piloted by the husband of a Nascar executive crashed into a suburban subdivision here today while trying to make an emergency landing, killing him and four other people and seriously injuring several others as at least two houses burst into flames this morning, officials said.

Nascar confirmed on its Web site that both people on board the Cessna 310 that crashed were killed: the pilot, Dr. Bruce Kennedy, a Daytona Beach plastic surgeon and husband of Lesa France Kennedy, a Nascar board member and president of the International Speedway Corporation; and Michael Klemm, a pilot for Nascar.

"This morning, at approximately 8:40 a.m. Eastern Time, a Cessna 310 registered to Competitor Liaison Bureau Inc. of Daytona Beach, crashed in a Sanford, Florida, area neighborhood," Nascar said on its Web site. At this time, we can confirm there were two people onboard, including the pilot, Dr. Bruce Kennedy, and Michael Klemm, a senior captain with Nascar Aviation. Both were killed in the crash."

This afternoon, authorities released the names of the others who died on the ground. They were Janice Joseph,

24, her son, Joseph Woodard, 6; and Gabriela Dechat, 4. They had been in the houses that ignited when the plane crashed into them.

Matt Minnetto, an investigator with the Sanford Fire Department, said the plane itself was scattered in several pieces across the area. Among the three survivors was a boy about 10 years old who had burns over 80 to 90 percent of his body, Mr. Minnetto told The Associated Press.

"It was an extremely intense fire," he said. The crash had spilled aviation fuel, contributing to the fire's spread.

Televised images of the scene showed huge balls of blazing orange flames licking at some homes and black opaque smoke rising high into the sky above the neighborhood. Neighbors said pieces of the exploding plane had landed on their yards and surrounding streets.

Various news reports, collectively, began to paint a word picture of what happened to my house and the neighbor's house.

The plane's cockpit filled with smoke, according to the pilot's last comments just before the plane crashed into my neighbor's house. A large portion of the plane where the pilot and passenger were crashed into the room where the young mother and her child were, killing them instantly.

The fuel tank somehow separated from the plane and crashed into my house, which is what caused the wall to shake. Within seconds the fuel tank exploded. That was the sound that led me to think there'd been a nuclear bomb possibly dropped on Disney World.

It would be about three years before I would learn the truth about how Jimmy and I got out of the house alive.

Publisher's Note: Excerpt from an email by Elaine Solis, Pete's step-mother's niece:

In loving memory of Gabi – July 10, 2007

Every day we hear it on the radio or see it on the news of accidents or fatalities that affect families around the globe. We are saddened by the tragedies of everyday life and empathize with families who have lost their mother, father, aunt, uncle, brother, or sister to such haunting memories which may fade in a week or so by other headlines, their names quickly forgotten.

Yesterday, the news I heard on TV hit so close to home. I was watching the morning news while Niko was playing and I saw two homes in Florida in ruins because of a fatal airplane crash around 8:30 a.m. Eastern Standard Time.

It was an attempt for an emergency plane landing as the plane was going mayday. The names had not been released yet but there were five fatalities reported, one being a young girl.

I was sad to hear of the news seeing the condition of the homes and the persons affected because of this emergency plane landing that resulted in the freak accident killing the victims.

Around noon when I was cooking lunch, I got a phone call from my mom. She was very solemn and quiet and had asked me if I heard about Pete's family in Florida regarding the plane crash. My heart sank to the floor. I had to find a chair as my mom told me that Gabi died and that Pete, Gladys, and Jimmy were in critical condition.

No other information was being released and the news was the only source of revelation at this point for family and friends. It happened to Andy's son (Pete), daughter-in-law (Gladys), grandson Jimmy (10), and granddaughter Gabriela (4).

The whole family was in their home when this happened in the early morning in Florida, not having a chance to flee unhurt from their home. So many thoughts ran through my mind.

I've met the family on a number of occasions before moving out to California. Gabi was learning to crawl and Jimmy was starting school before they moved (from Virginia) to Florida.

I was numb and couldn't believe what had happened on the other side of the country had happened to people I know.

Today in the news they actually released the names of Pete's family, and discovered also that a 24-year-old mother and her young son were among the fatalities (they were at home next door), and the pilot and co-pilot (died also in the neighbor's home).

Jimmy is in Cincinnati at a Burn/Trauma hospital and Pete and Gladys are in a Florida hospital.

Andy has packed for Florida as this will be a long duration (including hospitalization and recovery and rehab) for his son and daughter-in-law. I don't know if Pete and Gladys are conscious, or if they know that their baby girl is gone. I don't know if Jimmy is conscious, but the news of his sister hasn't been spoken of I would think.

They say that Jimmy's burns are very severe not including the long road ahead for this 10-year-old boy who not only has to deal with the psychological events of what has happened to him and his family, but is also fighting the increased vulnerability to infection because of his burns and rehabilitation.

My heart goes out not only to Pete, Gladys, Jimmy, and Gabi, but for the other victims and their families. I hope that Gabi is in peace and watching over her daddy, mommy, and big brother Jimmy.

In times like this, FAMILY and FAITH IN GOD are what make difficult times in life worth fighting for. It just makes me thankful for my family, my health, and living each day to the fullest.

As of yesterday, I learned that I may never get any more second chances in life ever again, so I'm going to do things right the first time. If I've ever wronged anybody, I'm truly sorry, and I will make it an effort to tell my family and friends that I love them because I'll never know if it will be my last. As far as holding grudges amongst anybody I've known, life's too short to be focusing on those grievances.

I've been looking at the pictures from Ofoto of Pete, Gladys, Jimmy & Gabi that my Tita had sent me from her trip to Orlando last fall. I can't believe Gabi is gone.

I know that Pete and Gladys will be missing out on Gabi's first day of kindergarten, first date, getting her driver's license, getting married and having kids of her own one day. I know that her spirit will live on within her mom, dad, and brother, and everyone who she's known and touched, including me.

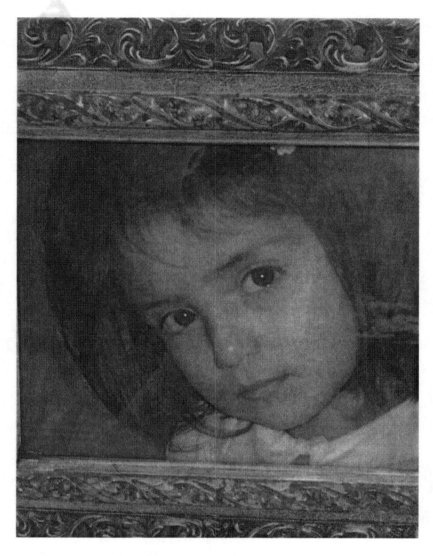

This is my favorite picture of Gabi. It was taken after being caught sneaking a Popsicle from the freezer by Gladys' uncle, who was visiting us in Florida. Because he made her put it back, she said, "That big boy was mean to me."

They thought I was toast

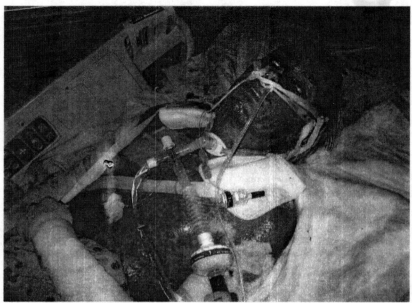

After the debridement, almost no skin was left on my body. The areas that were not burned are where skin was grafted and harvested for transplant.

People do not survive serious burns over 96 percent of their body. The lead doctor did not expect me to live, in fact they gave me 132% chance of dying. They take your age and add it to the percent that your body is burned and that's your chance of dying. My good friend and business partner, John Nootenboom, asked him, "How many people have survived injuries like this?"

"None."

"Well," John replied, "you got something to shoot for because he will be the first."

John really stood up for me. My immediate family was too wrecked emotionally to make any decisions. John took up most of the slack. He made sure my business affairs were taken care of; he interviewed, hired, and negotiated with the attorneys that represented us. He basically put his life on hold for months making sure things were taken care of for me. He is the unsung hero for me in this story.

Here's how John recalled the day of the plane crash and immediately after the coma was medically induced to try to keep me from dying from the pain. He heard the news on CNN.

> I remember going, telling your dad and getting your parents on the way. The next day I flew down. I met with your parents and Gladys.
>
> It was a zoo!!!
>
> Everyone wanted to be in the hospital and in your wife's room. Lawyers were popping out of the woodwork. I called Henry and his brother because his brother had been involved with a like accident. He said do not do anything for at least a month.
>
> No lawyers!!!!!
>
> One law firm with all the billboards got to Gladys so we had a meeting on day two or three at the hospital. Your parents and wife, to my surprise, asked me to take over, so I listened to the lawyers' advice then went to work getting rid of them. Gladys on day two had already agreed to see them and had signed one form which I later said we would SUE them because they sent a law student over acting as a lawyer – when she signed she thought he was a lawyer.
>
> So far you were just a pain in my butt.
>
> Then we had a meeting with the doctors and your family in the same room. The main doctor said you would probably die because your body wouldn't retain water. Then asked if we wanted to go see you.
>
> Everyone was very upset so they asked me to do it. As I walked down the hallway to see you I remember looking up at the ceiling and thinking *What, why . . . God, what is your plan?*
>
> I didn't want to see you like that but knew I had to.

Tim's assurance from God

My friend from grade school in Virginia, Tim, who gave me the Bible I left for so long unread on the coffee table, also wrote down some remembrances.

I believe it was about two years prior to the accident I received a phone call from you. You recently moved to Florida; we didn't talk as often as we normally would, so I was excited to hear from you.

After our normal greetings you said, "Guess what I'm doing?"

To which I responded, "What's that?"

You said, "I'm getting baptized!"

I was immediately filled with an enormous amount of joy. I wasn't expecting that because we've talked several times about Jesus and salvation. I recall your responses were always related to you having difficulty accepting it. At the time of those discussions, I wasn't a very good example of someone who was saved. So it made sense why you had difficulty.

But I knew when you told me you received Jesus as your savior, that it was real. You have always been a person of conviction and not one who just went for anything that came your way.

After we hung up I immediately called Emily and told her the good news. Through the motivation of the Holy Spirit I told her, "God is going to use Pete for some big things!"

The vision the Holy Spirit gave me was you reaching thousands of people worldwide. I kept seeing you standing in front of thousands of people.

Fast forward to July 10, 2007. My sister called me while I was at work. She said there was a plane crash in Florida, and, "You need to call Pete and make sure he's ok."

I told her I would, but I sort of laughed it off because I thought *What are the chances that someone I know would be involved in such a freak accident?*

At this time, we had no idea who was involved. I tried calling you a couple of times over the next two days and left several voicemail messages. You didn't respond, which was not uncommon, because I knew you were an extremely busy person.

On the afternoon of July 12, 2007 I remember pulling into my driveway and Emily came running out of the house in a hysterical state, tears pouring down her face. She literally met me at the end of our driveway. I didn't even have a chance to get the car to the parking spot.

Seeing her in this panicked state caused a million thoughts to go through my head. I thought *Something happened to my mom, one of my boys is hurt badly, the dog was run over* and on and on.

The first words out of her mouth were "Gabi was killed!"

In my disbelief I asked, "Gabi who?"

She responded, "Gabi Dechat!"

"What are you talking about? How? Killed?"

She told me the details your dad sent in an email to us with the subject "Tragic News."

From the information we had there wasn't much room for hope that you would live.

I called your dad to ask what I should do. In his wisdom he told me to stay home and not travel down right now. He knew you had a long road ahead, that eventually the people would fade and that's when you would need us most.

Although I didn't agree with him I honored his request.

The rest of that night I cried out to God, begging Him to save your life. I could not sleep at all that night. I was praying and reading God's Word, looking for something that would give me hope. Then the Holy Spirit spoke and He spoke loudly. He said, "Remember I told you I was going to use Pete for some great things?"

I said, "Yes."

He said, "Then why would I let him die? That would make me a liar and I am not a man that I should lie."

I ran upstairs and woke Emily up and said, "Pete's not going to die. God's not going to let him die."

I could see in her face she thought I was crazy; first for waking her up at 3:00 a.m. and second for saying something that seemed so far from reality and speaking it with such confidence. I reiterated what God told me, and Emily faithfully came in agreement with this Word.

Never in my life did I have such certainty, so I knew it was Him.

About a month after the accident I drove down to Orlando with your dad for my first visit with you since the accident. Of course, there was much talk about you, your recovery, and your future. I could tell your dad was being cautious to say you were going to get through this alive although he had some hope.

When we got to the ICU the nurses were hesitant to let me in to see you because only immediate family and clergy were allowed. Your dad said, "This is Pete's brother! You're going to let him in to see his brother, thank you!" And that was that. A black man going in to see his white brother.

Emily and I walked through the ups and downs of your time in the coma, getting calls on different occasions from your dad:

"They're trying to get Pete's body to accept food. His body is rejecting the formulas. He can't last much longer without food."

"Pete has a bad infection. He might not make it through the night."

"His body is rejecting the skin graft."

"Pete has a surgery coming up; the Dr. said this could kill him."

The amazing thing is I didn't worry. I put all my trust and faith in God and that Word the Holy Spirit gave me. I experienced firsthand the verse that says "...the peace of God, which surpasses all understanding, will guard your hearts and your minds in Christ Jesus."

I thought it was important for me to share with your dad what God told me and let him know you will live and your story was not over.

I believe it gave him hope.

Life Post-Coma

Then came the pain

The ambulance took me to the hospital on July 10, 2007. I don't know how many surgeries and other procedures were done to me while I was in the coma.

When I woke to Christmas music, I really didn't understand how much time had passed. It was also the first time I felt the pain of my injuries. I didn't know the extent of my burns, but the pain seemed to be everywhere. I literally thought all my toes were broken even though not one was. It felt like a needle was being stabbed constantly in the arches of my feet – it was the nerves waking up.

I had bandages covering most of my body because of all the open wounds. Not being able to see because of the scarring on my eyeballs took some getting used to, and they kept putting a salve on my eyes, which made it even more blurry. I also couldn't speak because of the tracheotomy. That was one of the greatest frustrations, not being able to communicate my needs. I felt cold, and the sheets were too heavy for me to move.

When the fire happened, I was physically very strong. I worked out bench pressing 300 pounds and could squat 500 pounds. Considering I was only 5'7 and 165 pounds or so, that was a lot. My biceps had biceps. Imagine my shock when I woke up from the coma and was not strong enough to move the sheet.

I had a lot of concerns.

Why are my joints freezing up on my right side?

Why is a tube in my nose?

I managed to touch my leg with my left hand. My knees were now the biggest part of my legs. I thought about how much work it took to gain that strength, and how long it would take to rebuild those muscles.

Another shock to find out I now weighed only 95 pounds.

One question everyone avoided answering:

Why is my wife not here?

I did find out why the tube was in my nose. It was how I got fed. The tube went down to my stomach. It kept coming loose so they sewed it to my nose.

I also knew that if I was to get out of that bed, I needed to start working to get out of that bed. I know God will be God, and He is always faithful to do His part, but we have to do our part too. I remember it was very early on I started doing crunches as best I could to start rebuilding muscle. A nurse walked in and saw me doing that and said, "You put me to shame."

During those first hours of finally being awake I processed these questions over and over, which was hard to do at times because of the pain. The pain would kind of ebb and flow. Sometimes it would be unbearable and I would just have to count through it, and others it would be just like a sunburn – like it was just there.

There was so much pain over so many parts of my body that I couldn't focus on it all. Some things that would normally have been awful if nothing else was going on, really were unnoticed because there were more intense areas of pain. It's really hard to explain in a way that someone could understand it.

Dad walked in. I could tell it was him by the unique sound his shoes made. His walk is unmistakable, even to the blind.

He greeted me as if I'd been awake the whole time. He was elated to see me respond.

But my muscles were so weak I couldn't move my mouth enough to mouth the words I wanted to say. Communicating was frustrating for me, and everyone else.

Three-week shifts

When I turned 18 and moved out of the house Dad and Mom divorced. But when I needed their presence the most they were there for me. Although still living in Virginia, they worked out a plan that they would come down to the hospital in Orlando, Florida and take turns staying with me in three-week shifts.

They said one of the first things I asked them to do was read from the Book of Job to me. I asked them to do this so many times that they got a recording of Job and played that for me.

Here's what my friend Tim wrote about the Book of Job:

> My last trip to Orlando was shortly after you were woken up from the coma. I remember walking in the room, holding your hand, and you looked at me and said, "The Lord gives and He takes away. Blessed be the Lord."
>
> To this day I consider those few words the most powerful and impactful words on my life.
>
> Then you asked me to read the Bible, specifically the Book of Job. You made me read the entire book in one sitting. You kept saying, "Keep reading."

That was months before my life became even more like the woes Job went through. That would be the biggest shock of all.

Brutal day-to-day grind

So many needs in the hospital. It was tough. If no one was there 24/7, those needs went unmet for a long time. When you're in pain, or drowning in your own phlegm, five minutes seems like hours.

When my mom was there, she slept in the room with me, which means she didn't get very much sleep at all. I was supposed to be rolled every hour or so, but I had lost so much of my muscle mass that after ten minutes the pain of my bone pressing against what little tissue was there became unbearable. I would beg her to roll me.

They got an air bed for me that would rotate me automatically. Sounds good in theory, but that mattress would deflate frequently, causing me to rest on the steel pipe frame that went down the middle. I had a bed sore on the back of my head, and on my sacrum – both resting on the pole when the bed deflated. The infection was so deep on the one on my sacrum that they had to cut part of the spine away. What was left was very sharp. If I bumped it, or even sat too hard, it felt like it would poke right through the skin.

I had respiratory therapy four to five times a night.

One time Tim spent the night there. The next morning he said, "Ain't nobody sleeping in here are they?"

Mom slept in the room even before I had the skin grafts, when the room was kept at 98 degrees because I had no skin. She was covered head to toe in protective plastic gear. She said she lost 25 pounds or so during that time.

I had one African nurse that was so good to me – I wish I could remember her name so I could find her and thank her. She washed me, and painstakingly scrubbed off the scabs that were ready to come off. She cared for me like I were her own son.

Because of this I also got in the habit of picking off the scabs that were loose. One morning John (my mom's husband) came to see me – he probably wanted to see my mom too. He looked at the floor and said, "Looks like you found some bacon bits." But he knew what it was.

I had physical therapy twice a day. This was brutally painful, but I was like *bring it on*.

There was only one male therapist who it was too painful for me to take. He wouldn't stop, even when I was crying and begging him to. I know he thought he was doing what I needed to have done. My mom made sure that was the last time he worked on me.

I was not allowed to eat or drink. They would only rub my lips with a sponge. My dad would slip me an ice cube when he could, but they could always tell somehow.

The first time they let me eat:

"Wow…oh boy, real food!" It was more like "Oh no!"

They let me have anything I wanted. I asked for cheese pizza; that I would regret. After about two or three bites, I threw up, and immediately aspirated my vomit. That was really scary. Think of the infection that could develop from that being in my lungs. And there was no one there with me.

I remember the first time I sat up. They pulled me up, and then I would fall back to being crooked. They said to sit straight.

"I am."

They pulled me up straight, but it felt like I was crooked. So I would fall back to what I thought was straight, which was like a 45-degree angle to the side.

Once I got past that, they would put me in a chair. I was supposed to be there for one-half hour. But I was so thin that I could barely make it ten minutes.

I remember the first step. A therapist was on either side of me, really holding my weight up. When I took the first couple of steps, I called everyone I could think of. Every day pushing it more. Then I got to the door. Eventually I got to where I could walk to the end of the hall. It was like running a marathon to me, but I loved the challenge.

That hole in my throat

One time, when I still had the trach in, some mucous partially covered the tube, and I spoke when I wasn't supposed to be able to. It was very raspy, but I could be understood.

EVERYONE working on the floor came in to witness that!

They had expected me to have a speaking valve reasonably soon, but certainly not to ever speak without it.

There were times when there was so much mucous in and around the trach tube that it was hard to breathe.

It was good when they installed a speaking valve on the trach tube. And it was a great day when they took the tube totally out.

All during the coma and for months afterward my body was like a tube depot:

The tube in my nose through which I got fed for several months.

Tubes in my arms. Very difficult to find veins.

Medicine port.

Foley catheter tube.

Gall bladder.

Tubes in my anus. I was given stool softener and hardener at the same time. Frequently it would clog up. Sometimes would go up to six days without passing.

Had monitors patched all over my body. Always fell off causing alarms to sound. There wasn't enough skin in many of the areas for the tape to stick.

Sometimes I would lie on the control. Dr. Smith was the main doctor for the entire floor. Saying that he was mad when he found me lying on the box was an understatement.

Daily procedures that needed to be done for my benefit still were very painful. For example, beside the therapy sessions, my bandages were changed twice daily. Would take about an hour each time. I was always glad when those sessions were over.

The fact that I could take steps was a miracle.

They thought I might never walk because the Dorsey flexor muscles were gone – these are the muscles that lift the foot up for walking.

Another miracle came after an attempted skin graft while I was comatose. Most of the skin grafts were already done by the time I woke up.

I was told they tried to graft bovine (cow) skin onto my chest. My body rejected it. The miracle was that my body unexpectedly started to produce "skin buds" – and the skin on my chest grew back.

What the therapist overheard

I remember sitting on the edge of my bed while Tim was visiting. I started crying and said, "I'm just sick and tired of being sick and tired. I'm tired of being in constant physical pain. I'm tired of always crying about Gabi. I'm just tired . . ."

By this time he was crying with me. He got up off his chair and just hugged me. That's when the therapist saw it and scheduled the visit of the woman who was lit on fire by her boyfriend after he poured gas on her. She was burned so badly that she lost both legs below the knees. She was the most impressive visitor I had.

Really showed me – if she is out there making it, I know I will. Thank God for your problems because you could have somebody else's.

I silently prayed, *Thank you, God, for this pain in my feet because it means I still have feet.*

That emotional outburst was the closest I came to a pity party. I got upset, sad, and even angry at times, but never felt sorry for myself. Only by the grace of God did I never once think *Why me?* I always thought of it more as *Why not me? Bad things happen to good people all around the world. Why not me?*

In John 21:21, Peter looked back at John and asked Jesus "What about him?" Jesus' response in verse 22 is harsh. Basically He said, "What's it to you?" It made me think *what's it to me if I suffer when others don't? Just walk the road I'm on, and don't worry about anyone else's.*

I know that's easier said than done, but if you can really live out the idea that "life is 10% what happens to you and 90% how you deal with it," it will be easier to try and take those thoughts captive.

One time in the gymnasium, I was walking and saw a man in a wheelchair. "What happened to you?" I asked.

"Got shot in the head."

"Don't give up. One day we'll be out there shooting hoops again."

No matter what's going on you can be an encouragement to others.

They didn't want me to know

While still in the hospital, close to my 37th birthday in 2008, I finally learned why my wife did not come to see me. Everyone tried to prevent me from knowing. They were afraid it would cause me to give up, or hinder my healing.

While I was still in the coma, she had decided to get on with her life with another life-partner.

To say I was devastated would be a severe understatement.

She'd been named my legal guardian.

In this book, out of respect for her privacy, I used the alias Gladys.

Because I had to go through her to get to see my stepson Jimmy, it was like reopening wounds. I loved – still do – Jimmy as if he were my biological son. He's a super young man. But I had to sever contact with her so I could get on with my own life. This meant I couldn't see him.

I miss him. I wish I could just tell him I love him and that I'm sorry for not being there for him. I wish I could've seen past my pain to help him with his. I wish I could ask him for forgiveness.

The rehab rollercoaster

I was in the hospital and three rehab facilities for close to five months after I came out of the coma.

One rehab experience was a nightmare. I won't name that place.

I remember my first night there, a big woman turned on the light and woke me up at 5 a.m. "Time to take out that foley tube." She then grabbed my penis in one hand, the tube in the other, and just yanked it out. Kind of like ripping off a Band-Aid real fast, but a million times more painful. It bled.

It didn't get any better from there.

At one point I had to tell them I had the right to refuse any care I didn't want to participate in.

They would have me roll on my stomach as part of my physical therapy. My wounds were still wide open on my forehead, and it would reopen the scabs that had formed. The sheets and pillows would be bloody after my sessions.

One night, the phlegm was so thick in my mouth that I was literally choking on it. I kept pressing the call button, but no one would come. I had to turn my head and try to push it out with my tongue. It dripped down my check and neck. I was so angry, I thought I was actually going to drown and die in that facility. I was able to swallow what was left in my mouth. Another night, I had to go potty, and again I kept pressing the button, but they wouldn't come. Eventually I couldn't hold it anymore. About 15 minutes later, a nurse came in and barked out exasperated, "What is it?!"

"Now it's too late, and there's a mess to clean up."

One time they clamped the foley tube to collect a urine sample – they forgot to unclamp it. It felt just like a urinary tract infection again. They took so long to respond, my dad had to unclamp it.

Because of the poor care, my mom threatened to sue them. They promptly asked if they could find me another place to stay.

The transition to Inova Mt. Vernon Rehab Center in Virginia was like ascending from hell into Heaven.

I flew there on a Lear jet. The nurse on the plane was so nice. We talked while en route and I told her how much I liked Triple Crown Jelly. She was so touched by my story that she ended up mailing me a jar of Triple Crown Jelly which I could only find at Maters and Taters fruit stand.

Mt. Vernon looked like a step backwards, but the care was 20 steps ahead of the previous place. Dr. Gisolfi a.k.a. "Dr. G" was fantastic. Everyone there was GREAT!

You'd expect doctors to be so serious, but Dr. G always wore crazy ties. He'd tell me about his ties having dancing skeletons or other crazy things to entertain the patients. He was a funny man who would actually listen to me and my concerns. I ended up seeing him for several months as an out-patient after my discharge.

My stay was supposed to be only three weeks, but Mom was in Europe for a month. They let me stay for five. I loved that place.

Jacara – She was the nurse I had a crush on. I remember asking her why she was so nice to me. She said, "I like you because you're nice, and you're funny." But I guess handicapped guys weren't her thing.

Some of the staffers I remember well included Kelly – PT, Carla – PT, and Stephanie Schwartz– my primary therapist. I did many more months of out-patient therapy and they were all amazing.

One thing that is invariably true is that we all make an impact on the world around us. Some of the most seemingly inconsequential things we do or say leave a mark that can last a lifetime. Stephanie left such a mark with me.

Typically, whenever a nurse or doctor said to me, "You're looking good" in reference to my healing, my knee-jerk reaction was to say, "It's hard not to look good when you're me."

However, that particular day I was lamenting about how anyone could be interested in me with all the burn scars. She stopped what she was doing, looked me square in the eye and said, "With your personality no one will see the scars."

Speaking about personality. I remember the first time I was able to wipe my bottom again. I mean, nothing is more humbling than having your butt wiped by anyone other than your parents. After my solo flight on the commode, I hobbled back to bed. I plopped down on the edge and started singing this song and doing a little dance:

"I wiped my butt, I wiped my butt.

Nobody helped me; I did it on my own."

My sister called – I sang the song to her. My mom called – I sang the song to her too. Pretty much anyone that I spoke to – I sang the song to.

It was a good day.

Even though they still had me wearing boots to prevent dropsy (when you can no longer lift your foot up), I started to get up and walk on my own using a four-post cane to go to the bathroom. One night, part of one of the boots broke off. When the nurse came in the next morning, she asked, "I wonder how this part of your boot got all the way over here in the bathroom? How do you suppose that happened, Pete?"

"I don't know."

I know what you're thinking: "You lied to her." But I didn't. I really had no idea how it *broke off.* I thought they were stronger than that.

"Listen, if you're going to walk, at least get certified first."

When I was being released from Mount Vernon, they wheeled me down (as is protocol) but I asked them to stop at the front door. I was determined to walk out on my own two feet. Dad snapped some pictures of it. My favorite is with my mom a step or so behind me, her hand over her mouth in disbelief. Tears of joy flowed down her face.

Auditioning with a frozen right arm

After playing heavy metal, and then jazz, I stopped playing guitar for many years. I became much more interested in exercise and sports as I moved into my late 20's. John Nootenboom was the one who got me back into working out. He wanted to get in shape and asked me to go with him.

My personality doesn't allow me to do anything half-hearted, so when I was in I was IN. The same thing with softball. An employee asked if I would join their team because they needed some people. I really didn't want to because I thought softball was a girl's sport. How wrong I was. I, almost embarrassingly, told Tim and another friend, Doug about it. I was shocked how emphatically they asked if they could come too. Before long we found ourselves on three different teams that all became competitive.

On one of the teams, we had a former pitcher for the Washington Senators. This was the church league team, and the field was short – only 270 feet. At the time, he was in his 70's and he could no longer hit the ball over the fence, but I remember one practice when he got close. The ball fell about 10 feet short. In his frustration he took a ball and threw it over that fence, almost effortlessly. I used to love his stories about when he played against some of the greats. He described Yogi Berra's hitting as a work of art. Because of my new found love of sports, I no longer had time for music.

The only reason I started playing bass again was because playing a musical instrument was recommended as good physical therapy for my hands. If I hadn't gone through the fire, I may have never started playing again. Tim would pick me up and take me to church with him. I remember the Sunday I brought my acoustic bass to church. I wanted to show the worship leader, Angela Donadio, at River of Life that I really could play.

I think at first she was just being polite listening to me play. But who can blame her? At that time, I was still blind, and my right arm remained frozen from my wrist to my scapula from the heterotopic ossification (extra bone growth). Additionally, I still needed a four-post cane to aid my walking and both my pinkies remained permanently contracted, making them unusable. I think it was much to her surprise that I could play well. And she invited me to join the worship team.

It was very difficult for me though. Because I was blind, whenever I had to play, they would make a CD for me. I had to spend about 30 hours a week learning and memorizing the songs. Everything was by ear, and feeling where I was on the fret board.

Learning to play again was very painful. My skin was thin, so pushing down on the strings, and plucking the strings, was a real test of mind over matter with the pain it caused. Also, with my arm frozen, I had to play with my right hand in an awkward position draped over the bass.

Surgeries and re-do surgeries

I had to have two surgeries on my elbow, and two on my shoulder, and LOTS of therapy to get the motion I have in my right arm. It's not perfect, but before the surgery, the elbow was completely locked in place, and the shoulder only had an inch or two of movement. It was a completely useless appendage.

The first surgery on each joint didn't work because the new *traumas* from the surgeries caused additional bone growth. They just froze up again. The second go-round, they gave me radiation treatments to retard any new bone growth that might come from the trauma of the surgery. Bingo!

Since I had picked up MRSA while in the hospital– a form of serious staph infection, my wounds healed slowly. I would frequently have active infections in the surgical sites. That's exactly what happened to my elbow.

On one visit, the doctor examining the wound stuck a Q-tip in the infected opening in my elbow. The Q-tip went in almost two inches before he said, "Maybe I shouldn't have done that."

The infection spread quickly, and I was back a few days later. It was so bad that one time when treating it, I bent my elbow to allow for a better angle so it could be dressed. The puss squirted out.

When the doctor looked at it again, I smiled and said, "It's pretty bad."

He couldn't believe it. "S***, I just stuck the Q-tip in it."

I was there so often, and my dad would get in line to sign in and register at the front desk, I would just walk to the back. "Come on Dad" and that became the norm, just walk right in.

From the second shoulder operation I developed a huge hematoma. I mean big. I joked with the doctor that he was going to have to create a bra for my shoulder. It took several weeks but eventually went away.

The No. 1 doc in his field

When I went to see the corneal specialist it was very early in my recovery. I still had to be rolled in on a stretcher. This doctor was one of, if not THE doctor, that perfected the cornea transplant. When he first looked at my eyes he said, "I'm sorry, there's nothing I can do to help you."

"What do you mean?" I was shocked.

He started to explain that even if he did, my eyes would end up drying out and I'd lose the eyes anyway. That my corneas were too thin and too damaged to even try.

"You are the best in the world!" I said. "If you can't help me, then who can? Listen, I have 20/800 vision. I'm blind. If I lose the eye, what have I lost? Try one eye – pick the worst – it's my eye, let me take the risk. If it doesn't work, it doesn't work."

Can you believe he consented?

You know it's the favor of God when you can convince the world's foremost specialist to change his mind.

I needed multiple surgeries to prepare my eyes for the cornea transplant though.

They had to plug some of the tear ducts to help keep the moisture from draining out. Part of my lower eyelids were removed and sewn onto the upper eyelids so they could close completely.

When I was finally going in for the transplant, one of the nurses was asking about my accident. He said that this transplant would be the least painful of any surgery I will have had.

My first thought when I woke from the surgery was *he lied!!!*

Why would I have thought cutting the front of my eyeball off, and stitching a new one on with 18 stitches inside would NOT hurt?

One of my favorite sayings is "It beats getting poked in the eye with a stick."

Well this was exactly like getting poked in the eye with a stick.

The surgery went well, and every visit he would ask the fellows and other doctors if they knew my story. I think I'm a walking textbook for many in the medical community. Every visit there would be four or five people examining my eye.

I have a light sensitivity. Bright lights make me sneeze. Staring directly into those bright lights, and not moving, was on par with sitting for my nose surgery – I'll tell you about that in a minute. Harder was not moving while they were sticking the scissors in to cut the stitches, or when they pulled them out with tweezer-like utensils – with the bright lights right in my eye.

To convince him to do the other eye took more than two years.

He kept telling me he was perfecting a new procedure. One visit, as he was admiring how well the eye was doing, I said, "I can't wait till you are saying that about the other eye."

"You really want me to do it, don't you?"

"Of course I do. Who else can? You are the best in the world!"

For a second time, God's favor fell upon me. He consented.

It also turned out wonderfully.

Just so you understand, the vision took years to come back. Finally, when I got my first pair of glasses, I could see. Now my vision is 20/25 with my glasses, 20/20 with a special hard contact. Getting the hard contact in and out was very tough for me, so I prefer to wear the glasses. You know, I never really knew exactly what my wife looked like (oh yeah, that story is coming later too) until that first moment I put the glasses on.

Sometimes you have to just sit and take it.

I briefly touched on my nose surgery. As a burn victim I experienced extraneous bone growth in my joints that had to be excised, and skin tabs that had to be cauterized off. I was having difficulty breathing because I couldn't clear it out. I went to an ear, nose, and throat specialist as I suspected more extraneous growth.

This was a young doctor, and what I remember most was his Bostonian accent. I loved it – like *wicked cold* kind of accent, like Cliff from *Cheers*. It was great. He examined me and said, "That's not human tissue in there. Looks more like burlap." He tugged at it a bit, but it was attached and not coming out. "We're going to have to schedule you for surgery."

"Wait, Doc. I'm here, you're here. Let's just do this."

"No way" he said "The nose is the most sensitive part of the body. I can't just numb it like at the dentist. This is a serious surgery, and I don't have an anesthesiologist here today. I don't want to start and then have to reschedule it because you couldn't take it."

"Look at me. With what I've been through, you will never find someone with as high a threshold for pain as me."

As insane as it was, he consented.

"At the first sign of pain I'm stopping."

I sat stoically in my chair, focusing on keeping my face completely expressionless. The doctor gave my dad a bowl to hold under my chin as he advised me to keep my mouth open for the blood to flow out. "Don't swallow the blood because it'll make you nauseous."

He made the first cut with his scissors. The sound to me was as if he were cutting through construction paper. My white tee shirt quickly became not so white. The blood flowed out so fast that much of it splattered out of the bowl onto me. I don't know exactly how many cuts it took, or how long the surgery was. My focus was on not showing any reaction to what I was feeling.

He pulled out a two-to-three-inch bloody mass. It turned out that a compress was put up my nose and forgotten about at some point before I was out of the coma. This was now more than a year, maybe even two, since the accident. It had been left in so long that my body had grown around it.

"Wow! You really didn't feel that!" he said in disbelief.

"Are you kidding? That was the most painful thing I'd been through in my life! I just couldn't let you know or you would've stopped."

He fell back in his chair. If he was in disbelief when he thought I couldn't feel it, you can imagine his disbelief knowing I DID and didn't show it. "You were right. I've never seen anyone with that threshold for pain."

Pursuing Mrs. Right. The one I thought got away.

Since my wife left me, I had nowhere to go when they could no longer keep me at the hospital or in rehab. The cost of my care I was told was around $6 million, so I understood at some point I would have to leave.

But I was still blind, unable to walk, bathe myself, feed myself, or dress my open wounds. I asked my mom if I could stay with her until I got back on my feet. She was my best nurse anyway. Not figuratively, literally; the nursing staff gave her an award when we left.

Of course, she said, "Yes."

My best friend Tim would drive one-and-one-half hours every Sunday to be at Mom's house by 7 a.m., and then drive back one-and-one-half hours to take me to Sunday school and worship service at church. We would hang out all day, go to the evening service, and then he would drive me home around 8 p.m. He spent six hours every Sunday driving me.

One Sunday, we arrived a little late to class and the discussion had already begun. Bob Dickens was the class leader and had just asked a question. I don't even remember what it was. All I remember was the angelic voice that answered. When you're blind, all your other senses seem to be more acute. Smells and sounds were more distinct. But it wasn't only the sound of her voice, it was what she said:

"Like I tell my children, the mitigating circumstances have not changed..."

I think Tim blurted this out, but everyone tells me that I did:

"You talk to your children like that?!" In an accusatory manner.

The entire class burst out in laughter.

I thought *I have got to meet that woman. She sounds so intelligent and sophisticated.* I fell in love with her voice.

But in a church of 500 or so, a blind guy that doesn't walk well has little chance of finding anyone. So I thought I missed my opportunity as the class dismissed to go to the worship service. I solemnly limped my way to the sanctuary as Tim led me. After service, I made my way out the doors of the sanctuary. Then I heard that sweet voice of the one that I thought got away. Not only that, she was talking to ME!

It turns out, her cousin was burned at a very young age. Because of this, Judy had not only been used to being around a burn victim, she wrote a paper on the care of burn victims. She started asking me questions about my care. She was standing with a recently-divorced friend, and somehow got to "When you're old like me, you tell your body to do this and it can't anymore."

To which I replied, "What are you, all of 26?"

Keep in mind I was blind, so I had no idea what she looked like, or even a guess as to how old she was. We all laughed.

Then I said, "Does that get me brownie points?"

She replied, "I didn't know we were keeping brownie points, but yes."

I could tell by how quickly she said she had to go that I might've embarrassed her. I yelled, "Wait, I didn't even get your name."

She said, "Judy."

She did not realize I was blind. I could see shapes, so I knew roughly where the eyes were and always looked there. She later told me how much of a gentleman she thought I was because I didn't check her out the way other men did. I always looked in the direction of her eyes. In this way I say I was blessed with being blind. Consider Romans 8:28:

> "And we know that all things work together for good to those who love God, to those who are called according to His purpose."

No one will deny that bad things happen. The question is whether you have the patience to allow God to prove this scripture true in your situation.

I had no idea how beautiful she was. But it wouldn't have mattered anyway. Time takes the looks away from everyone. If that's all you're in love with, you will be very disappointed later on. I fell in love with her, proposed, and married her not fully knowing what she looked like. I fell in love with what mattered, her heart.

When I got in the car with Tim I asked, "I can't tell, but she's cute, isn't she?"

Because his kids were in the car he answered, "I'm not at liberty to say."

"I knew it, she is."

Some time had passed, and I hadn't run into her for a while. My friend John Nootenboom invited me to go with him to Charlotte, North Carolina on a business trip.

Driving back through the mountains, I was thinking about Judy, wondering if I'd ever talk with her again.

I pulled out my phone. It had a voice mail. Can you believe it was her? She had gotten my number from the church and was inviting me to share with the Spanish ministry. She is Puerto Rican, but I didn't know it because she had no accent.

When I got home I called. I was very nervous, and she sounded nervous too. After she asked if I would share, I said, "Yes, but will this involve lunch and maybe some nice conversation?"

She laughed and said, "Yes, but later."

We talked many times over the next week. One of the things she said she found attractive was my smile. I said, "You can have one just like it too. It's porcelain." She couldn't believe it.

During one of our conversations that first week I told her matter-of-factly, "You know, one day I'm going to marry you." Yes, you read correctly I told her I was going to marry her in the first week.

She thought for sure she would scare me off and she tried. She told me how she was a single mother of three, but, when that didn't work she told me how she homeschooled. That didn't work either. What's funny is these very things she thought would scare me off, made me love her more. I thought *How selfless. She could do anything she wanted, but she's sacrificing her wants for her children.*

That Christmas I proposed – a very thought-out plot. I had many accomplices, and we invited our closest family and friends. There was a box inside a box, inside another box, inside still another box. Each layer had a personalized message, a pillow embroidered with "I love you, Judy"; a ceramic plaque saying "forever and ever"; a set of glass cups – one saying "All the things I want" and the other saying "to share with you."

The final box was a beautiful, wooden ring box. And like the jokester I am, I got down on one knee and said, "I hope you like this."

I opened the box and it had a little plastic ghost ring from a vending machine. The real ring was in my dad's pocket. She handled it with class, but later told me how she hated that.

Judy and I married on July 28, 2009 in the backyard of the house I bought for us to live in.

We drove off after the wedding in a 1982 Rolls Royce we had beautifully restored just for this occasion. My dad was our chauffer. About 10 miles down the road, it started overheating. Turned out the "Just Married" sign on the grill blocked all airflow causing the overheating. We ended up being driven in the minivan.

When we returned from our honeymoon I moved in with her to our wedding house.

Author's comment: I believe you will enjoy reading in my wife Judy's own words what her thinking was from the time she first encountered me.

How I met the Love of my Life

I had gone through some major setbacks and was very discouraged. I found myself suddenly alone, barefoot and pregnant, being dropped off at my parents' house. I had two toddlers, two and three years old, and one on the way. I was now a single-mom facing many challenges.

Fast forward seven years.

I was being prayed for and told, "The time of just enough is over and God is saying abundance . . . Eli is coming with the camels."

I had no idea what that meant. Frankly, all I needed was grocery money and help with those emergencies that come up unexpectedly. In the fall of 2007, at a special church event, I went up for prayer and told the preacher, Randy Clark, that I was just burned out and discouraged. I did not know how I could keep going. It was a sad pity party, but my pain was real, and I was truly overwhelmed.

Something very unusual happened.

He motioned to the first row of seats and we sat down to chat. That should've been the first sign that something strange was about to happen.

Who does that? And besides, there was a long line of people waiting to be prayed for by him.

He told me what his life was like before he had an encounter with God where he was transformed. He said that it resulted in a lifestyle of peace and stamina that he experiences daily.

I was excited. I thought *Yes, that's what I need! Bring it on. That's a prayer I can believe in. Here he is sitting down to chit chat about this. He obviously knows what I am talking about and what I need.*

Right?

And then he prayed . . . for a helpmate?

Did he just pray for a husband?

I think I remember saying a silent objection to Heaven.

I kept my head bowed and my eyes closed, but I was having a totally different conversation with God. *I thought he got it. I thought we settled that I was overwhelmed. I didn't need someone else to care for. What is he thinking?*

He continued to pray. He asked God to bring me someone with a gentle spirit, one that would help me with the weariness of motherhood, and who could share the burden.

I always try to hide my initial reaction and process whatever is being said, and boy I sure hope I hid what I was thinking as I walked away. Inside, I was shaking my head in total disbelief. I think that there was a small part of me that admitted I needed help, but my pride kept me from fully embracing that prayer.

In the following months, the theme continued.

Either a word spoken over me or a feeling while I prayed, but marriage seemed to be the common thread. I went to many people to run this by them and ask their opinion. One by one, they expressed joy for me. I kept asking more and more people, trying to find someone, anyone, who would assure me that that was a prayer that needed to be rebuked.

I couldn't.

Everyone I mentioned it to was genuinely happy for me.

When I shared it with my pastor, he too was happy for me. I explained that I didn't want to get married. Very sternly he shared that if God had to forewarn me, it was because my heart was not in the right place. He went on to explain that I had to change my attitude or risk losing out on the blessing that God was sending my way.

Ouch!

After that I decided to stop my search for a sympathetic ear. But some of my friends who I had already talked to about this continued to give me marriage advice, and buy books about relationships for me.

One in particular, Anita, who was going through a divorce, even advised me to write a list of what I wanted in my husband. I explained that if I went down that road it would be telling God that I was ok with it, and I wasn't. She tried to reason with me that if God was going to do what He was going to do, I might as well ask Him for what I wanted. So, as I read the books and heard the advice, I decided that I would write important points down.

It was interesting because what happened in the coming months was that I felt God pouring out HIS love on me.

One time in the summer of 2008 I was in my little closet deciding what to wear that day. I felt myself surrounded by a cloud of the most amazing love I had ever felt. I was unable to remain standing and just bowed down crying. There are so many things in my life that made the simple act of deciding what to wear a real struggle. I never wanted to be noticed. In that moment, I felt God telling me He wouldn't judge me, and that He loved me just because of who I am. I wrote in my journal,

God I know this is weird, but I can't take your love much more. I feel your caresses, I feel your kisses, I feel your embrace and it makes me so much more aware of the void in the here and now.

May your unfailing love come to me, Lord. Am I crazy? I think that you're doing this on purpose! I think you're showing me your goodness and just making me hungrier for more intimacy. I can't believe it. It's almost like you're doing a bait and switch for my benefit.

Taste and see that the Lord is good. I think I can see how the enemy is attempting to sabotage me. (I didn't want to admit I wanted to get married. I was resigned to singleness but I felt a real emptiness.) *So please, Lord, even as I think you're going too fast and that I'm not ready yet. Lord, please, don't let this be a long journey – but not my will, Lord – but yours be done!*

Little did I know that by the end of the summer I would meet my future husband. It began as a seemingly uneventful encounter.

I was burnt out and could never see myself waking up extra early to make it to Sunday School. It was only an hour earlier than the main Sunday service I was already attending, but an hour for me as a single mom of three was just overwhelming. Things changed when they announced that there was a new class being offered and that the teacher was an astronomer. Then when they announced that it was a family Sunday School class it was a done deal. I made plans to have a dry run the week before it started to see how early I would have to wake up to make it to church in time for class.

Well, I managed to get the kids ready and actually get to church on time. What I had not planned on was that I'd be in church an hour early with no class to attend. I grabbed the brochure – yes, brochure of the Sunday School classes as they had so many that they published a booklet listing them. I tried to zero in on one that I'd be interested in even if it was just for the one class. After scanning the list, I decided on *The History of Israel*. Seemed interesting being that my family is said to have Sephardic roots. I was so happy I actually made it on time and even had time to greet some friends.

The class that day touched on Nehemiah 22, Balaam's donkey. I made a comment that it seemed the prophet kept going to God to see if He had changed His mind, and that it reminded me of my kids. You know, when kids keep asking the same question expecting a different answer when nothing's changed. I said, ". . . and I tell my kids, the mitigating circumstances haven't changed..." Before I was done with my comment I heard the biggest chuckle coming from the other side of the classroom. A man's voice said, "You talk to your kids like that!?"

This just got everyone laughing, including me. But, I had to offer a rebuttal. "Well, it's a proven fact that whatever level vocabulary you use at home is what your children will use later in life."

It didn't matter. Everyone was still laughing and the class moved on. I was just a bit perturbed. I was so tired the last thing I needed was a run-in with the class clown. I was glad when the class was over and without much thought to the exchange, I went on my way.

Our church has about 500 congregants. The church is divided into three vertical sections as you face the platform. I happened to be sitting almost to the back of the first section as you walk in. I pride myself in being a good audience member. I have to admit though, it has something to do with being raised in an old Spanish Pentecostal church where you were pinched very hard if you couldn't sit still. Imagine my horror when several rows ahead of me, sat a man who seemed to be *trying* to distract the preacher. I wish I could say he had ants in his pants but it would be an understatement.

Oh how it ruffled my feathers. He sat right in my line of sight to the preacher and I just kept praying. I thought for sure it was going to be the end of me. I couldn't concentrate. This man just kept shaking, almost as if he needed to go to the bathroom. He did this throughout the entire morning service. I was so relieved when it ended, I just wanted to get my kids and go home.

Instead, I bumped into my friend Anita – the same one that told me to write a list – and called her over to say "Hi." When I saw the new church member that had been in a house fire, I asked her to go with me to talk to him.

When I met Pete Dechat, his arms were covered in large scabs and keloids, which were more like mountain ranges. I immediately wanted to know about the treatments he had undergone, about medical advancements in skin grafting, and about the awful process involved in debridement (the surgical removal of dead tissue).

As a child, I spent a summer with my Godparents, and their daughters. I especially spent time with my cousin Gladys who was closer in age. The fact that she was scarred from third degree burns around her neck and shoulders did not even faze me. She had many operations from skin grafts to releasing of scar bands, but it didn't bother me. To me she was just my cousin. The time I spent there had a great impact on me and I carried those memories with much fondness.

Later in life I wrote a paper about burn victims and the scars they carry in their hearts. I wrote about how, unlike other injuries, the injuries of burn victims are ongoing in the sense that they undergo skin grafts on perfectly healthy skin enlarging their overall scarring. Which also adds trauma to their self-image.

I just wanted to keep talking to him and ask about his personal experience. His friends Tim and Emily joined us when suddenly Pete said something about how I look young for my age. I just giggled and he asked me if that earned him brownie points. We all started laughing.

I realized this was the class clown from Sunday School and the guy with the ants in his pants. Try as I might to keep the words from coming out, my mouth blurted out, "I didn't know we were keeping brownie points, but.... sure," I said with a smile.

What was I thinking?

I'd dodged the ball for so long, what the heck? I was so embarrassed. I just wanted to run and hide, which is exactly what I did. This time I couldn't even get the words out as I ran away, excusing myself to get the kids from children's church. All I heard was Pete calling out to me, "What's your name?"

"Judy," I yelled back without stopping.

I had no idea that the prophecy prayed over me by Randy Clark was unfolding right before our eyes.

For over eight years I kept my eyes down, not interested in anyone and sent out the vibes that said

"BACK OFF, BUDDY" very loud and clear. I really couldn't believe that I flirted back with a total stranger. Why did I say that? Who said that? There's no way I did that. It was like witnessing an invasion of the body snatchers with someone else controlling what I was saying. I just went home and paced like some high school girl with a bad crush. The whole week I practiced how I would react if I bumped into him. I literally acted out various scenarios: a hand wave across the parking lot, passing by pretending not to have noticed him, acting as if I didn't remember his name.

I was a wreck.

And when Sunday arrived, it might as well have been Judy's comedy hour. I scurried about trying to avoid him seeing me. I had butterflies in my stomach and lost track of where he was on the property. After rushing my kids out of their class, I almost bumped right into him on my way out of the children's building. Startled by his presence, I just said, "Oh, hi!"

Really?! All that rehearsing and all I said is "Oh, hi!"

What I didn't know was that even though I was two feet in front of him, he was blind and wouldn't have known that I was passing by.

His blindness was a blessing in disguise. He didn't look at me as some men look at women, and that allowed me, as a rape victim, not to immediately put the walls of self-preservation up. I was able to enjoy talking with him because I didn't feel the usual vibes I got from other men.

He later told me he recognized my voice immediately and how happy he was that I said "Hi" to him. He also explained that he seemed to have ants in his pants because some of his joints on his arms were locked due to extra bone growth and there was no way he could scratch himself. The only relief came from scratching against something, in this case, the church pew.

I guess God was making sure I noticed him.

It wasn't long before I knew I was head over heels for him. I couldn't remember the last time I allowed myself to feel pretty. One Sunday morning, I stood in my little closet and put on my brand new white summer dress and twirled around looking forward to seeing Pete. I was in love! My friends later laughed about how "Judy was trying to look good for the blind guy."

Coming from a conservative Spanish family, I felt obligated to tell my father about Pete before it got back to him from someone else. When I told him I thought I was in love, he said, "I thought I noticed you smiling more. So who is he?"

I went on to explain how we met in church and I figured I should prepare him for what Pete looked like.

"Well, he walks with a limp and the help of a four-post cane. He has an elbow locked in place and bandages on both arms. He has several bald spots. He's blind and he is burned from head to toe."

"Is this a joke? Are you serious?"

"I'm serious, this is not a joke."

"Is he a Christian?"

"Yes."

"That's all that matters. Now, how did that happen?"

I am thankful that God also honored my prayer from the summer of 2007 when I asked him not to allow this to be a long journey to marriage.

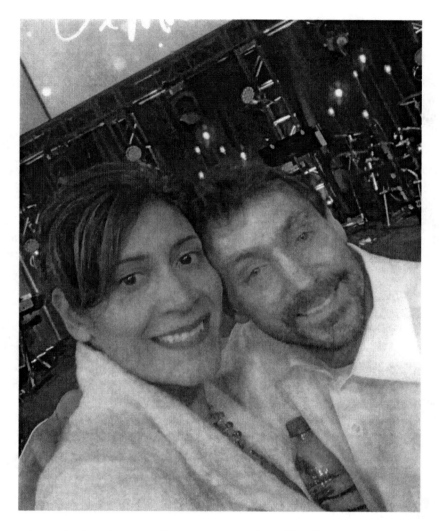

Judy and I just before playing at our church's Christmas night of worship concert. I'm lucky this one didn't get away.

Coffee concoction

I really love coffee. You can tell, because part of the story about the plane crash is that I didn't even get to take my first sip when it hit. I drink coffee every day. I've really been enjoying it lately with cinnamon, cardamom, and a dash of cayenne pepper.

Judy never drank coffee before meeting me. That was a big joke that she didn't even have a coffee maker. She was the *social* coffee drinker and sometimes drank coffee while she was out and about.

I brought the coffee maker into our relationship.

I totally corrupted her. Since I used to work for Schwan's Ice Cream, I used to make it with ice cream every day instead of milk or creamer. Add to that whipped cream, caramel drizzle with crunchy sugar sprinkles and voila, instant bliss.

Starbucks had nothing on me.

Even people who'd never liked coffee loved my creation.

After I saw the video, *Is sugar the new fat?* I drastically cut my sugar consumption.

Judy was an unintended victim of that decision.

"Sure, now that you've got me completely hooked on your coffee, you're going to stop! I've been hoodwinked!"

To us a child is born

We eventually moved from the house where we were married into a larger house that we over-renovated. The rule of thumb is supposed to be to own the cheapest house in the richest neighborhood. We did ok on the first part, but got carried away with the remodeling. What I also didn't count on was that they started to build tract houses in the neighborhood. Not only did we overspend on the remodel, but values dropped.

Double ouch!

The house does hold special meaning for us though, and it's not just to exemplify the mistakes we've made. This is the house where our baby was born.

A year after I proposed, Christmas 2009, Judy gave me a memorable present – a pregnancy test showing that she was pregnant.

God was giving to me more than I could have dreamed to ask for. Early on, Judy decided she wanted to have a home birth. We took the Bradley method birthing classes, got a midwife, rented a birthing spa, made a plan complete with assistant coach to help me because I was going to deliver the baby. We were ready.

One thing we didn't do was see whether it was a boy or a girl. Everyone was certain it was a boy because of the way Judy was carrying. There was no reason to deny my father-in-law's request to honor the baby as he was sure it would be a girl. He wanted to name her Rebekah. He was so happy when we told him he could. We even picked out a middle name, Louise, in honor of Gabi.

Between Judy and me, we had already picked Timothy Andrew, in honor of my best friend and my dad. Judy's mom had a dream with me holding a baby boy with blue eyes just like mine, and we were certain it was a boy.

Two weeks before the baby was due, the midwife wisely said that I should be prepared just in case she isn't able to get there in time. This was going to be Judy's fourth child after all. She thought it might come quickly.

We practiced with a baby doll what to do if the baby had the umbilical cord around its neck, delivering the placenta, and so on.

The contractions became intense and consistent. We called everyone and waited, and waited, and waited some more. The baby didn't come.

We sent everyone home and apologized for our baby so rudely standing us up and not coming.

A week later, about 5 a.m., Judy started having intense contractions again, but they were not very consistent. Judy constantly said, "This isn't it." She decided to get in the birthing spa, figuring we paid for it, we may as well use it.

Suddenly, she got up and ran to the bathroom. I kept timing the contractions. They seemed pretty regular to me, but Judy insisted it wasn't time. She got up from the toilet. "I thought I had to go, weird." Just as fast, she said she DID have to go and sat back down. This happened several more times. For those who don't already know, feeling like you have to go is one of the signs that the birth is imminent. I told her we should call the midwife, but Judy wanted to wait for a more decent hour before we called.

This was about to change. Sitting and standing was like doing squats which helps speed the birth.

"You should call, I feel the head."

She waddled back to our birthing spa and climbed in.

I woke the kids and called everyone. The midwife was two hours away, but had an assistant that was closer.

By the time that the assistant got there the head was already out. This poor woman was nervously wringing her hands. I was calmly helping Judy breathe and encouraging her. Her mom later said that if it weren't for my calmness she would have lost it.

I was in the spa with her and had the privilege of delivering the baby. You should have seen, and heard the surprise when I announced, "Welcome Rebekah Louise." Her first pictures are in black-and-white as all we had was baby blue clothes and blankets. It was a wonderful surprise, and my father-in-law finally named one of his grandkids.

Paying it forward

The house we live in now was built to be our *forever* house. Judy and I designed it with what we as 80-year-olds would need. We really loved doing it. Every nook, bathroom, and light fixture – every fit and finish – was designed, picked, and procured by us. There were other great minds involved, of course. But the bulk of it was designed and decided on by us. Our contractor, Karl Mosier, performed a miracle because the plans were three total pages. I don't think there are many people who could have done what he did.

At one point, he told us we weren't allowed to go on the Internet, read any magazines, or go on vacation anymore. His least favorite phrase became "I have an idea..." because that meant a change was coming. He was great though. Even though his knee-jerk reaction was usually "It can't be done," the next day he would come back with a solution.

The entire process was long. We had some terribly expensive mistakes. One such mistake was that our huge, arched windows for the front of the house came in too big. There were fingers pointed from everyone at anyone.

Bottom line, we ended up purchasing the replacements out of our own pockets. $10,000 worth of windows useless. Or were they? They sat on our property for a year. I wasn't going to throw them away. I paid for them. I was going to find a use for them.

Our good friends, Mike and Cindy Zello, were starting Beauty For Ashes, a Teen Challenge home for women who struggle with addiction, and their children. I know what they do is effective, and had been supporting the men's Teen Challenge for years.

Beauty for Ashes was to be only the third such facility in the country, and the first on the East Coast. God blessed them with the building, but it was in need of a total makeover. It would've been the perfect candidate for the extreme makeover home edition show. God worked miracle after miracle to renovate that building, and my windows became part of it.

They had three large windows that were damaged and needed to be replaced. My two giant, expensive mistakes were not going to be for nothing after all. Those two windows look like the two stone tablets for the Ten Commandments in that house. Praise God that even our mistakes don't go wasted.

There are too many other miraculous stories of how God provided for this center that an entire book could (and should) be written about it. But I want to share one that I got to witness firsthand. The cabinets were just installed, and Mike and Cindy were picking out the countertops. They could only afford the lowest grade counters available. I told them to hold off while I reached out to our granite guy, Roni from J & A Custom Granite. He's done a lot of work for us over the years, and he is not good – he's great. I remember one day I drew a design for a granite pass-through on a napkin. It had a very decorative shape and edge; nothing straightforward about it.

The next day it was installed just as I wanted it. So when I asked him to go and measure for BFA, I told him I would be paying for the counters. It was to be my donation to Beauty For Ashes.

He informed me that he had watched me for years bless other people. He and his wife had been praying for a way and the opportunity to be a blessing the same way he watched us be. This was their opportunity. They donated the granite countertops.

That actually made me cry. You never know how your actions will affect the people around you. They weren't even the direct recipients of a blessing from us, but our actions still impacted them to pay it forward with the blessings God has given them.

Straight-talking John

My mother's husband, John Rathbone, passed away in May 2017. John was strong in his faith. I will see him in Heaven.

John and I did NOT have a great relationship. But he loved my mom and made her as happy as I've ever known her to be. Because of that I really did love him. He was very hard on me, and came across as very rude – even insulting at times. But he had the courage to say to me truths that no one else would say.

When I went to live at my mom's, the wound of my wife leaving me was still very fresh. I was visibly letting the wound fester. It showed in conversations with others.

One day John sat me down at the kitchen table and let me have it. "Those so-called friends that keep talking to you about Gladys are no friends at all! They're killing you, and you need to stop it!"

Ouch!

As I think back about it, it was true. How can you ever get past the past, if you keep living in the past?

As a man thinketh, so is he.

I was dwelling on something that was dead – my marriage former – and was letting it kill me along with it. That's when I started to think about the future and not the past. I wasn't healed immediately, but the healing process could now start in that area of my life.

Another time, my pastor had all the fathers stand in recognition of Father's Day. This was the first Father's Day after the hospital and rehab. I could not bring myself to stand.

Was I even a father anymore?

Tears rolled down my cheeks as I sat there. *How can someone be a father if their only child was gone?*

When I got home, I asked my mom for a hug as I cried and told her about it. She cried with me, then went upstairs.

John came down shortly thereafter. In typical John fashion, he sat me down. "Listen, your mother tells me that you're not sure if you're a father anymore. Of course you are a father! You will always be Gabi's father. My daughter died in a car accident when she was 16, but I'm still her father just like you're still Gabi's father."

Wow!

Talk about what I needed to hear when I needed it. Think about it – she's in Heaven. I know I'll see her again.

There was one much less serious moment that I have to share.

John loved to watch MSNBC and drink his wine every night. His favorite spot to do this was right where the bed was set up for me. It was in the basement of their three-level townhouse. They finished it themselves, and it was amazing. John really was amazing with his craftsmanship. Where I might be Harry the homeowner gone bad, he was Harry the homeowner done right.

Mom would sponge bathe me and dress my wounds while he did his evening routine. He was very liberal in his views and enjoyed watching MSNBC. I'm very conservative in my political views. I think he thought of me as a Neanderthal.

Anyway, one night he got up to use the restroom while Mom was taking care of my wounds. Now in their house, they had a rule that everyone sits using the bathroom. No standing to pee. So out of the bathroom we hear "Uh oh, we have a leak, Monika."

Now you have to imagine that with every sentence his voice was getting louder to match his alarm. "Oh no! It's a bad one!"

"Oh no! It's pee – wait, it's me! I'm peeing on the floor!"

I laugh even today as I'm typing this.

When he was dying, we were all there. One of his daughters, my mom, my sister, and I. It was 12:55 p.m. I know because I called the time. I'm saddened when I think of him, all the wasted time and emotion. You never really know what you have till it's gone. But I'll see him again too. He was devout in his faith and love for Jesus, so I know he's in Heaven now.

Just like the rest of us, he had his faults, but I am so thankful for him having been a part of my life.

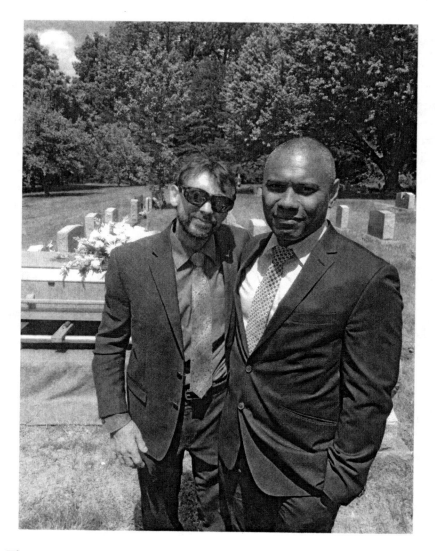

This is my best friend Tim and I at Straight talking John's funeral.

What I learned from a horse

I wasn't raised on a farm, or around farm animals. Closest thing to that for me is when my friends would go *cow-tipping* (at night when the cow is asleep knocking it over).

I bought land that was close to the church, and close to my friend Tim. I liked the idea of having some privacy, so we started with 15 acres. I continued to grow that to where we now have 47 acres.

When Tim asked me if I wanted a couple of horses, I jumped at the idea. I had no fence, no barn, and no knowledge of how to take care of horses. Frankly, I had no business at all getting horses.

But Tim told me of a man fighting cancer and could no longer take care of his two horses, Shaka and Pepper. They were beautiful.

We immediately had someone put up a fence and build a lean-to for shelter. We have since put in a barn, hay barn, chicken coop and pen, and divided the field into several paddocks.

I love having these animals, but they sometimes teach you lessons through the pain of loss.

Horses are big, strong animals. Shaka was about 1,100 pounds, so I had no idea how fragile they were. Pepper started rolling around one day as the season was getting colder.

I didn't know what was happening, but when she started to get lethargic, I called some horse people to help me understand. They were alarmed by my report of her flopping around and said to walk her nonstop until they got there.

By the time they got there it had been dark for two hours. It was cold, and I was struggling to keep her on her feet. The vet showed up shortly after they did. I had never heard the term *colicking* before. I didn't realize this is life-and-death for a horse.

The doctor explained everything going on with her, and that because of her flopping around, her intestines got twisted up. I learned that horses cannot throw up, so all the food was stopped up causing her great pain. For us, constipation is an inconvenience; for a horse, it can be a death sentence. This poor horse put her head to the ground, and fluid started to drain out of her nose. The vet, and the horse people that came to help, both told me that she had to be put down.

I couldn't believe how deeply I was hurt. I cried as if for a child. How is it possible to love that deeply so quickly?

I called the couple that gave the horses to us so they could say goodbye. One of the most difficult calls I've ever had to make. They came and cried with us. They cut some of the tail hair to keep. I thought that was a good idea and did the same.

Since horses are herd animals, everyone suggested getting another one so Shaka wouldn't be lonely. Tim's next-door neighbors also were horse people, and so they brought one of their ponies over to keep him company.

Enter the picture, Dudley.

Dudley was too smart for his own good – like Houdini of the horse realm. One day, this too-smart-for-his-own-good pony really lived up to that.

He broke into the tack room and ate about 75 pounds of feed. That day his owner was scheduled to come with a farrier. When she got there, she walked in on Dudley lying dead in the stall with Shaka trapped behind him.

At this point, we had several goats, so I decided I wouldn't get any more horses.

Three weeks before I wrote this, Shaka, who was now 31 years old, stopped pooping. We right away got the horse doctor over knowing how serious it was.

A year earlier, the same thing happened. We put him in an intensive care horse hospital and he got better. Because we caught it so early this time, we didn't think that would be necessary. We had that vet over almost every day for two weeks, and he still eventually lost that battle.

We had to put him down.

I sat there with his huge head in my lap crying like a baby.

How did this happen?

We caught it, we were doing everything right, and still couldn't help him get through it. I had a hard time seeing through my tears as I strapped him to the tractor to move his lifeless body.

A friend that works for me saw that I had moved him and asked if I did it by myself.

"Unfortunately, I've learned things I wish I didn't have to know owning horses."

I have part of his tail, too, and brought part over to the couple that gave him to me.

Shaka was such a constant. I could always count on him waiting by the fence for me when I'd drive back home from anywhere. It really forced me to realize how much I took him for granted. Seeing him yell at us for food from the edge of the fence, how many more times would I have gone over and given him a treat, or just pet him, had I known how little time left I had with him.

Do you hear that sound?

That's regret. The same regret I felt when my mom's husband John died. I regret taking him for granted.

It caused me to think about what else – or more appropriately, who else am I taking for granted?

I immediately thought of my dad. This man that took me to every doctor appointment; this brilliant man, who now as he's aging, is forgetting more than he used to know. Many memories rushed through my mind. We may not have had much of a relationship when I was growing up, but oh how I realize how much I love him now.

My dad was a toddler in WWII Austria. He knows what it means to do without. So now he is, let's call it *thrifty* (cheap), when it comes to tipping.

I moved in with Dad after a particularly rough run-in with my mom's husband, John. I had stayed out later than he thought appropriate (10 p.m.), so he was yelling at how much of a spoiled brat he thought I was – not in front of me, just loud enough so I could hear it. So I moved to Dad's.

Dad wanted to take me out to eat. The VFW was having $2 dinners, his treat. With the two beers he drank and the two dinners, I think our tab was a whopping $10.

I said excitedly, "Dad, give her a $10 tip."

"Are you crazy?"

"Dad, do it," I encouraged. "That $10 isn't going to change your life one way or another. But wait and see what it does to hers."

My first wife was a waitress, and I've heard plenty of stories about tippers. Some good, but many more bad.

When the waitress saw the tip, her eyes bulged out of her head in disbelief. Her sincere gratitude and that great big smile – even I, the blind guy, could see it. I nudged Dad. "Worth every penny isn't it?"

"Yes it is," he responded a bit emotionally. "Yes it is."

Dad was extremely tough on us growing up. But once I started to prove myself as a young adult, a lot of my stupidity from adolescence was forgotten. He treated me with a great deal of respect and deference. Our friendship was forged in that deep mutual respect for each other, despite our personal shortcomings. I count him amongst my closest of friends. It really is like the love Paul describes in 1 Corinthians 13.

1 Corinthians 13:4-7 New King James Version (NKJV)

[4] Love suffers long *and* is kind; love does not envy; love does not parade itself, is not puffed up; [5] does not behave rudely, does not seek its own, is not provoked, thinks no evil; [6] does not rejoice in iniquity, but rejoices in the truth; [7] bears all things, believes all things, hopes all things, endures all things.

He didn't recognize me

Three years after I was an in-patient at Mt. Vernon, I went back to visit the hospital staff, especially Dr. G. I walked up to him. He was standing right in front of the room I was in.

He didn't recognize me.

I said, "That's my room there," pointing.

He still had a poker face.

When I told him my name, he was so stunned that he took a literal step back. The look when the realization hit him that it really was me standing in front of him was priceless.

That I looked so different and improved that he did not at first know who I was, really made my day.

The angel has a name

Today's culture celebrates the imagined, the contrived, and the made-up. We look to heroes like Superman, Batman, Thor, Captain America, Iron Man — the list goes on and on – to be our role models.

What we rarely discuss, or more accurately, what we ignore, are the real life superheroes:

The military, police, and fire fighters.

I ran back into my burning house because of the love I had for my Gabi. My actions were not heroic. They were really selfish. I wanted to save my daughter. I ran into harm's way just as much for me as I did for her.

But someone else ran into my house, not knowing any of us. That was truly heroic. He didn't do it because he was going to have the Grand Canyon-sized hole in his heart like I now have from Gabi's death. His motivation to save us was selfless and without regard for his own life. This hero I speak of is Ryan Cooper. He is the fire fighter that was able to help Jimmy and I get out.

I have to take you to the beginning of this part of the saga.

From the time I woke from the coma, many eye-witnesses said Ryan wasn't there. He was widely being hailed as a hero on TV and in the news, but many people were telling me he was a fraud.

Looking back, I can't believe how foolish I was to give any credence to what these people were saying. Their stories of how events happened did not at all line up with my own very vivid memories. For three or four years I believed what these people had told me as true – that he was a fraud.

Then one day my worship leader called me. I was on vacation and was driving through Florida at the time. She asked me to tell her the story again, so I did.

She said, "I think I'm reading your story on a Firehouse Subs cup, but it's talking about a Ryan Cooper."

I was so mad. "He's a fraud. He wasn't even there! I can't believe it!"

When I got back home, I was still upset. A friend of mine, who is leaps and bounds smarter than I am, said, "Why don't you confront him about it? If this is the most monumental event in his life, and it's a lie, the most loving thing you can do would be to free him from it."

I came up with excuses. "I don't even know how to reach him."

"Well, why don't you call the firehouse where he works?"

I thought to myself *Because that would make too much sense – duh!*

Still, more excuses flowed out:

"That was years ago."

"He probably doesn't even work there anymore."

I'm really quite embarrassed thinking of my cowardice at that moment. I'm not one who usually backs down from a confrontation.

What was I afraid of finding out?

As is so often the case, fear of the unknown – let's just say fear in general – is paralyzing.

Was it better to live with contrived stories than the actual story?

No!

I immediately googled the fire station that he worked at, got the number, and called.

They told me that he no longer worked there (as I thought), but instead of saying ok and hanging up, I said, "Someone there might still know how to reach him. My name is Peter Dechat, and he was the one that got me out of a fire when an airplane crashed into my house."

Everyone in that area knows that story, so there was no doubt he knew my name. I gave him my number, and just told him I had some questions.

When I hung up, I was certain that was the end of it. I mean, why would a fraud call up to be confronted and proven to be a fraud, right?

Not more than five minutes later, my phone rings with a Florida area code.

I knew it was him.

Now, my personality is kind of shoot first, ask questions later – not something to really be proud of, and I think God is helping me with that.

When I answered the phone, I didn't act like that at all. "Ryan, I just have some questions because no one's story really matches with mine. Can you tell me what you remember?"

He said, "In person, not over the phone. Too many people are trying to discredit me. How do I know you are who you say you are?"

"I understand, but I now live in Virginia, it's not like driving across town. Just tell me one thing. Everyone keeps trying to tell me Jimmy jumped out of his bedroom window. I know I saw him running down the hall. There's no way he would have run back into his room because right below it was where the plane's fuel tank hit. No one would have run back into that fire."

He paused for a second. "Now I know you are who you say you are."

And we started talking. He shared what he remembered, and his story was the only story that lined up with mine.

He told how when he went into the house, he found Jimmy first. He said he found him very close to the front door, but walking the wrong direction. He said he was doing the *mummy* walk. He said this is common with severe burn victims.

After getting Jimmy out, he went back in and ran into me by the steps (which are more than half-way toward the back of the house). The steps were also directly across from the master bedroom door. He said I was also doing the *mummy* walk and walking the wrong direction.

As he started to help me get out, he said he saw daylight through the ceiling. Keep in mind that we were on the first floor of a two-story house. If he was seeing daylight that could only mean everything above it was either gone, or soon would be.

He said he yelled, "Get out now!!" as he pushed me toward the front door.

Those three words "Get out now" stopped me in my tracks. Those were the words I said earlier that I thought was an angel, and what snapped me to.

I told him I didn't remember being carried out. He said, "It wasn't like superman. I didn't carry you out, I pushed you out."

He said my skin was melting off of me and coming off all over him. I realized he WAS there, and he DID get me out.

Before too long, I also realized that the call was more for him than for me. He was telling me of his struggles, his grief, everything he had to fight through since the accident.

I asked, "How do you deal with it all, are you a Christian?"

He said, "Not anymore."

At that moment I knew I had to meet him. "I am coming down, but you have to promise you'll come to church with me."

There was a very long, uncomfortable silence.

"Hello, you still there?" I asked.

"I am. I don't like it, but I'll go."

I took the whole family down. I wanted to see my former pastor, so I set it up. Unfortunately, the small church where I became a Christian was closed down. But he worked it out with the pastor of the church he was now attending that I could share my testimony there. They were so new that they were meeting at an elementary school.

When we arrived in Florida, we went straight to Ryan's house. When he opened the door, he was shocked. He said, "I knew I saved your life, but I thought what kind of life could you have after those injuries?"

Rebekah was only one or so at the time, and seeing her with my beautiful wife and me, I could understand his shock.

We spent time together, went to the Firehouse Subs headquarters and met the owners. It was a great time.

When we went to the church service, the pastor just let me have the entire service to share. Anyone who's been in any church for a while knows that's unusual. Pastors are typically very protective of the pulpit, understandably so because you wouldn't want some nut spewing out anything contradictory to the Gospel.

I shared and got to publicly thank Ryan for saving me. That had to be vindicating for him since many were treating him as a phony. I couldn't see well enough yet to see any tears, but I could hear in his voice that he was touched.

The pastor afterwards thanked me profusely for all the people we brought with us.

"What are you talking about? I only brought my family and Ryan."

The pastor said there were twice as many people there as normal – about 60 or so were there. I asked some of the visitors why they came today. More than one person said, "I don't know. I was just driving by, and something told me I should stop in."

The fire station Ryan worked at was very close, just down the street from the school where the service was held. We stopped by and Ryan introduced me to the firemen there, maybe six in all. When I shared how God saved me, they all laughed out loud.

After their laughter subsided, I quietly asked, "Ok, you are all professionals, right? You've all seen burn victims before, right?"

They affirmed both statements. "With me being burned 96%, what chances do you give me to survive?"

Everyone was quiet.

"You can't explain it. The doctors can't explain it. I CAN explain it. I didn't save myself. Why is it so difficult for you to accept that God saved me?"

No one tried to refute what I was saying.

"God saved me so I can share with people like you. People that would recognize the improbability of my survival. What more proof could you possibly need?"

As I was leaving, one of them came up to me, shook my hand, and said, "Keep doing what you're doing."

Ryan asked lots of questions about my faith, and how he could incorporate the Bible with the life he enjoyed living. I told him that's between him and God: Ask Him, He'll give the answers if you're sincerely seeking.

He told me at some point before I left that he thought I was the most influential person in his life at that time. That was incredible to me considering I only spent three or four days with him.

I cautioned him, "Hold on, I am no one's example. I can only point to the One that is my example. My relationship with Jesus only makes me better than what I'd be without Him. Anything you see worthy in me, worth commending, that's Jesus. Everything you see in me worth condemning, that's the real me. A relationship with Jesus doesn't make you perfect, just better than you'd be otherwise."

One of the most powerful things he said to me the entire trip:

"I may have saved your life then, but you saved my life now."

Miracle or lucky?

People sometimes want to dismiss the incredible miracle God worked in my survival, and they replace it with being *lucky*.

According to the doctors, I would have a better chance to be struck by lightning and survive – twice!!

Even if you wanted to go the lucky route, let's add up the luck:

I was lucky that a fire fighter lived one street away.

I was REALLY lucky that he just got home in time to actually see the airplane crash.

I was REALLY, REALLY lucky that instead of putting his protective gear in the station, as he said was customary for him, on that day he threw it in his trunk.

That's just the luck of him being there.

Not to mention defying the odds of the 132% chance (according to the doctors) I had of dying.

I'm hoping you can sense the sarcasm. Kind of like the Marty Simpson t-shirt: "Sarcasm is my love language."

It really does take more faith to NOT believe in God than it does TO believe.

My Testimony.
My Ministry.

Tim's vision
becomes a reality.

Pastor Yousaf set me straight

When people used to ask me about my ministry, I would always say, "I don't have one. I'm just a guy that loves Jesus."

Then a pastor from Pakistan, while visiting in Virginia in 2015, made two comments that impacted me.

Pastor Yousaf told me, "No, your testimony IS your ministry."

He also told me, "Most people think there are only four Gospels. Not true," he said. "There are five: Matthew, Mark, Luke, John – and yours. Many people won't listen to the four Gospels in the Bible, but the 5th Gospel – what Jesus has done in your life – that gets their attention."

He wasn't talking about my testimony specifically, but all of our testimonies.

I believe that statement is corroborated in Revelation 12:11. "And they have overcome him (Satan) by the blood of the lamb, and by the word of their testimony..."

Pastor Yousaf's boldness in preaching the Gospel reminds me of the Apostle Paul in the Bible. That is why I call him "Pakistan's Paul."

His boldness has been a source of encouragement to me right from the start. He has been threatened, and beaten. He says, "My days are numbered in His book. No man can take my life until that time. I'm not going to stop."

Why I am alive

As you have read this far, you know I believe that God brought me through the fire. And I believe He did this for a reason:

To prepare me to tell everyone I can about Jesus, who is the only way to experience eternal life in Heaven.

As Jesus said in John 14:6, "I am the way, the truth, and the life. No one comes to the Father except through Me."

I know this is a harsh reality that billions of people flat out refuse to believe.

This world is so depraved, and like lemmings, running full speed off the cliff to its destruction. The enemy is having a heyday, and many in the world do not understand what they are bringing upon themselves.

So, yes, I feel a very strong sense of urgency to tell people what their options are about where they will spend eternity after their physical death.

You never know if the person you're talking to today will be alive tomorrow. My accident was July 10, 2007. I didn't think when I woke up that morning I would never be able to hold my daughter again. Every day is someone's day to meet their Maker. I want to help make that a joyful meeting for as many as I can – not a regretful one.

When I gave my heart and life to Jesus, my soul belonged to Him. It was not just lip service. But I didn't become on fire for the Lord until after the plane crash and waking from the five months of coma darkness.

Jesus said two things that make me want to witness to people at every opportunity:

1) "Therefore go and make disciples of all the nations..,"
2) He also said, "If you love me, you will obey my commands..."

I do it out of my love for Him. I want to give Him back all that He deserves. I want to see His kingdom increase. Most of my adult life I worked in sales, and I was exceedingly successful. If I'm willing to work 16 hours a day talking to people about ice cream or blinds. I can certainly talk to people about Jesus. What you talk about the most shows what you are most passionate about.

This is my passion.

It's exciting to be able to see people in the differing cultures. What I've come to realize is no matter what the country, we have more in common than not. We all love, we all hurt, we cry and we laugh.

Most of all, we all need a savior, and therefore we all need Jesus.

There used to be a song. "We all want to change the world, but we don't know what to do..," You change the world one heart at a time.

I never think about the crowns that I'll lay at Jesus' feet – only my own. I go not for what I will receive, but for what I've already been given.

Every life saved through receiving Jesus is worth celebrating. What's most exciting is the *compound interest* that occurs spiritually – like the stone hitting the pond, the ripples reach the farthest edges of the pond. All the great evangelists – someone was the first to share the Gospel with them. I can't wait to see what the totality of the impact will be. If one of them will be the next Billy Graham or Ravi Zacharias, for example, that would be fantastic.

Go Team Jesus!!!

Foster children

My first mission trip didn't involve me sharing my story at all, but was an important step because it helped me to see outside the bubble I lived in. A group of friends were going to Hope of Life in Guatemala. The thought of going to a foreign country to be the hands and feet of Jesus excited me. And I was not disappointed.

This ministry bought an entire mountain that they built a hospital on, housed neglected elderly people, rescued orphans, and even had a home for special needs children called Kelly's House. This became my favorite place. Being able to love on these who are most often forgotten and left to die brought me a sense of joy and love that I had never known.

One of the families travelling with us was the Foster's. Yes, we went to Guatemala with the Foster children too, hence the title of this section. This family is amazing. I joke with Kip, the father that I want to be like him when I grow up. His wife, Maria, would eventually go on the trip with us to Cuba which I will cover in the next segment. Both the girls play on the worship team with me now. Sarah, the eldest, plays the piano and Lydia the violin. I wouldn't say it's angelic when they play, but I think the angels might actually stop and take notes from them. The girls and I led worship every night, and then we met to debrief and plan for the following day.

One such night we were told that we were called upon to do some painting. Lydia and I were the only ones that seemed excited. Because of this, they put us by ourselves in a group, and everyone else in the other group. Ten of them against us.

I quickly assessed the situation, as competitive as I am, and said, "This is totally unfair......You are grossly outnumbered two to ten." Luckily for them, our plans were changed and they were spared the utter defeat they would have been handed.

What I really learned there was how much greater a blessing it is to give than it is to receive. We went to pour out on them, but I felt that what I received impacted me more then what I left with them.

Hot summer in Cuba

My first trip abroad to share my testimony was to Cuba in August 2015.

Pastor Herrera is a presbyter in Cuba who was in the States visiting my father-in-law, Eliezer Rivera, who is an evangelist, as they were planning for him to visit Cuba. He stopped by to introduce us to Pastor Herrera. In a matter-of-fact way, he invited me to also make a trip to Cuba and share my testimony. I didn't even really take it seriously. Kind of like, "Let's have lunch sometime." But to him when he asked us to go to Cuba, as soon as we said "Ok" it was written in stone. We decided to all go together; Eli, Maria Foster, who is of Cuban descent, and my family.

We have nothing to complain about. Those people walk for hours in 100 degree, 100% humidity Cuban heat just to get to church. They packed into the back of semi-trucks like sardines to attend the meetings. You know there was no a/c in the back of the semi's or in the church.

The people there are beautiful and loving. They made a huge banquet for us at every meal, although they had to procure the food illegally. Judy eventually caught on that the reason they weren't eating with us was because they were waiting for us to finish so they could eat whatever was left over. We later found out that everyone has food ration cards. They must've all been pitching in from their rations in order to feed us every day. Their generosity humbled us. Our appetites were much smaller after we figured that out.

Their church was built by faith.

They didn't have any tools, not a hammer or a shovel. And they built it themselves borrowing what they could from neighbors. It is solid concrete, sagging just a bit in one of the corners. It is maybe 100 feet by 60 feet with a second level, wrap-around balcony. There is a terrace on the roof with somewhat of a kitchen, and a separate room where they had a beautiful banquet prepared for us.

The pastor told us that after it was completed, the government came to check out the church one day. "Very nice, we'll take the second level."

The pastor told them, "No."

They said, "You either give us the second level, or tear down the church."

Pastor said, "Fine, tear it down."

The government official actually relented and backed down.

Coincidentally, Pastor Herrera was in our area in the States while I was still writing this book. He was raising funds for his ministry as he does every year. It is always such an honor to have him visit.

Oppression and possession in India

My father-in-law Eli had a contact from India that he introduced me to several years ago, Pastor Rajan.

When that pastor heard about my story, he was touched and asked if he could name his orphan ministry after my daughter, Gabi.

I said, "Fine."

After a few more visits from him to the U.S., he invited me to share my testimony in India. Even in January when Eli and I went, it was in the 90's. Because I can't sweat on large areas of my body, I have to be careful so I don't overheat.

India is mostly Hindu. I was told they worship 33 million gods. I was blown away at the number of idols that were on display everywhere we went. There was a heaviness, and it wasn't the heat and humidity.

After one conference, while still praying for people, a pastor grabbed my arm and asked me to follow him. Toward the rear of the grounds they were praying for a man they believed was demon possessed.

I had never personally seen this, but I believe the Bible and I believed it possible for people to be possessed. When I arrived, the young man was crouched there as if he just ran a marathon, sweat pouring out of him, breathing deeply with his eyes still closed.

I thought I'd just place my hand on his head to bless him. As soon as I touched him and started praying, he contorted to this completely unnatural position and his face grimaced with anguish as if in great pain. I guess there was no language barrier with the spiritual forces.

I immediately started rebuking the demon. This man was bent over to where his upper body was parallel to the ground about 18 inches off the ground-*backwards*. I put one hand under his back because I was thinking he would fall, not that I was supporting much weight. I don't know how, but he didn't fall down.

I was in disbelief of what I was experiencing. But I continued to pray fervently with several others for him. After a long period of time – maybe six or seven minutes – a pastor threw water in his face, literally slapping him to snap him out of it.

When he came to and opened his eyes, he had a bewildered look about him, looking all around as if he was asking what happened without using any words. He abruptly took off – to where I don't know.

Were we successful? I don't know. I just know it was real.

I have never felt love like I did in India. They had constant processions, with horns and timbrels. They showed honor, and served us as if we were royalty.

This is where I learned what it meant to host someone.

This is where I learned what it meant to serve others.

But one thing I was shocked about was the way that wives were treated. It didn't even seem like a friendly relationship, but rather more of a servant/master relationship. They asked me to speak in front of 80 pastors. The message God put on my heart to share was Ephesians 5:25 – "Husbands love your wives as Christ loved the church..."

It was a hard message to that group. I actually apologized to Rajan if I had offended anyone. He said, "This is a message we needed."

There was only one older man that approached me. He said, "This is a hard lesson for us. I am not sure we are ready for it."

I said, "Yet."

One of the most memorable parts of the trip is when Rajan took me to the land I helped them purchase to build the orphanage. It was five hours south from Cuddalore, where Rajan lived. That is five hours at the crazy speeds they drove. It probably should have taken much longer.

Street laws may exist, but no one follows them. So coming 80 miles per hour to a red light at a congested intersection, they don't stop. They slow a bit, and honk constantly:

"I'm coming through, get out of my way!!!"

Absolute chaos, yet they have fewer accidents – at least what I saw while I was there – than we do here. My father-in-law was holding on to everything, bracing for impact the whole ride. I slept much of the way.

When we finally arrived, the villagers had a procession for us, giving each one of us a lime. I tried not to take it because I knew they were giving to us out of their lack, but Rajan said it would offend them.

There they unveiled the monument they put up for Gabi. It was black marble with her last school picture perfectly engraved into it. I cried uncontrollably, and most of the men cried with me.

Unforgettable. Simply unforgettable.

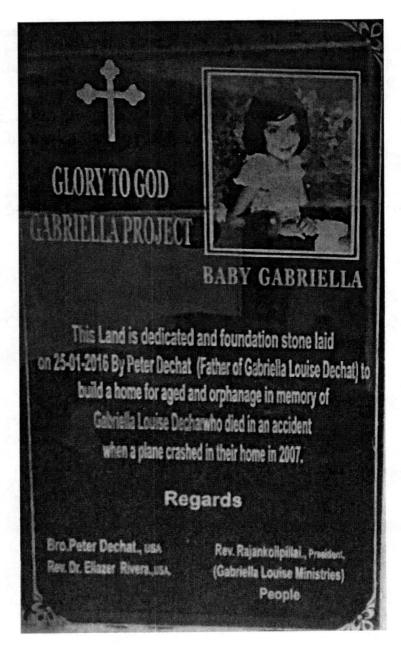

This is the monument Pastor Rajan surprised me with in India.

Ghana surprise

It always amazes me how opportunities arise that allow me to share my testimony to people in other countries. How I wound up in Ghana in June 2016 is a prime example. Although it was a surprise to me, it was not a surprise to God.

I was invited to play with the worship team from my old church, and it was there that I met Rev. Dr. Stephen Wengam, the guest speaker. After the service, we spoke and after hearing my testimony, Pastor Wengam looked at me. "I never speak like this – you can ask him," pointing to the man hosting him, "but you are to come to Ghana, and God will show you what to do when you get there."

"I guess I'm going then."

After Pastor Wengam got back to Ghana, arrangements were made for my visit. When I was leaving for the airport, my daughter Beka came running out crying. While she was handing me a little stuffed animal, she was saying, "Daddy, this is for you to remember me. Don't forget me, Daddy. I will never forget you."

She could barely get the words out because she was crying so hard. My heart melted as I gave her a big hug. Makes me want to cry thinking about it. That's the beauty of young kids, you can feel their sincerity.

I used that little stuffed animal when I shared my testimony in Ghana. I asked the people, "Do you know what this is?" holding up the stuffed dog. I then shared the story of how she gave me that toy.

"My daughter is the apple of my eye. What would cause me to travel 4,000 miles away from the ones I love the most? I came for you, as Jesus came for all of us. We are all the apple of His eye. He left the perfection of Heaven to come to this fallen world because of His love for us. So we wouldn't be lost. Why did I come? I came, because He came."

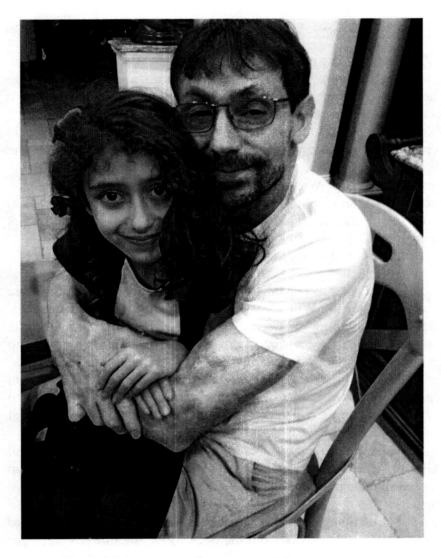

The apple of my eye. My Beka.

I had no idea of Pastor Wengam's prominence and importance. Not only was he a mighty preacher and pastor of a fairly large church and had a radio show that aired every morning, He was also one of four pastors that traveled with the president of Ghana.

When I arrived in Accra, the capital of Ghana, I was met by government employees. I was taken right from the plane into state cars, then to the VVIP lounge (very very important people) while all my entry paperwork and customs were taken care of for me. I stayed with Pastor Wengam, and was treated like family.

He had me on the radio four or five mornings at 5:00 a.m. I thought *Who is going to hear us that early?* But after I shared, he took calls – astounding, not just the number of calls, but how touched people were. He originally said I'd be on for one or two days, but after every day he said, "I must have you back tomorrow."

After one morning, he drove me straight to another radio station. This was a secular station. They were so touched they asked me to come for a second interview.

Another morning, one caller wanted to wish a happy birthday to the Chief Justice. After we went off the air, he drove me straight to her house. She told me that my coming was the best present she could have been given. She had been listening to us every morning on the radio. I prayed for her and her husband, and she invited me to share at her formal birthday service at her church. It was full of dignitaries. Even though I only had five minutes, it was still quite an honor.

Even my wife was ministered to back home. She listened every morning as well on the computer. She shared with me how for the first time she realized that God had redeemed even the name of my ex-wife. Her cousin who was burned as a young child had the same name as my ex-wife. She said God showed her that NOTHING is lost in His kingdom.

The pastor videoed me sharing as full an account as I could remember at the time, and transcribed it to be handed out as a tract. They said they handed out thousands of them.

My favorite story from this trip was the Muslim woman visiting the church one Sunday. The only reason she was there was because he invited her after she interviewed him. She "just happened" to pick a Sunday when I shared to visit. After the service, she invited me to share my testimony for her morning TV show. But the highlight wasn't being on TV. It was sharing with her personally during our recording session. She was visibly moved while I shared, at one point burying her face in her hands.

When I stopped, I saw tears running down her cheeks. "Is there something I can pray for you about?" I asked.

"My relationships," is all she said.

"No," I pressed. "This is your time. What specifically do you want me to pray for?"

"For my relationship with God and His Son."

I verified. "You want me to pray for your relationship with God and His Son Jesus?"

"Yes," she said through her tears.

So I prayed with her as she accepted Jesus into her life.

Then I prayed for the cameraman for his needs, and her assistant for hers.

This woman was now beside herself with joy. She said over and over again, "I can't believe it. You've made my day! Thank you! Thank you! Wow!"

Getting to Pakistan

We had known the pastor from Pakistan for several years by the time we went. We met him at an Awaken The Dawn Conference in Fredericksburg, Virginia. My wife dragged us all there as she had been attending these meetings for several years. She also invited my father-in-law to come.

We were all tired and cranky, really just a bunch of sourpusses. My wife was finally giving in and agreeing to go home when someone got on the microphone to recognize out-of-town guests. One man stood up from Lahore, Pakistan.

My father-in-law froze. "You won't believe this," he said. "The Lord told me to pray for Lahore, Pakistan. I didn't even know where it was. I had to look it up. I'm going to stay now."

He eventually brought the man from Pakistan to my house. His name is Yousaf, the one I told you is the Apostle Paul of Pakistan.

My father-in-law took a trip to preach in Pakistan. He told me, "Nowhere in the world have I felt love like in Pakistan."

At the time I didn't get it.

Five years later, Yousaf was here raising funds for his ministry, JDMN (Jesus Disciple Ministry to Nations). I hosted him, and tried to set up speaking engagements at local churches. He asked Judy and me to come and share my testimony in Pakistan.

We set out to start the process. Mind you, this is the Islamic Republic of Pakistan. The letterhead he sent the invitation on to take to the embassy has his ministry's name in bold print on the top. His email is kingjesus4me. It expressly stated all the Christian conferences, baptisms, churches to be dedicated, and so on. He wasn't trying at all to hide what we'd be doing.

We were turned away twice by the embassy. They weren't thrilled we were there, and we felt it. But the third time was the charm. We got the visas! We celebrated, took lots of pictures and sent them to Yousaf. That was Thursday late afternoon 4:30ish.

The next day, Friday, I was scheduled to play at a night of worship at my church; the power was out at the church though – and only on our block. Most places near us still had power. I told everyone, "I've been seeing this all week. It's a spiritual battle. Let's pray!"

We prayed, and we prayed. About 10 minutes before the worship service was scheduled to start, the power came on. The night of worship was amazing. I got back home at 10:30 or so.

One part of info I hadn't mentioned yet is that our flight to Pakistan was in 10 days. That is critical to keep in mind when you read the next sentence. I found my passport completely shredded on the floor, including the visa I received just the day before. My young German Shepherd had chewed them terribly.

I screamed louder than I had ever screamed before. I called my wife and said, "I guess we're NOT going to Pakistan!"

I was too upset to even cry. Beka's was damaged too, but you could still read it. Mine was trashed, and Judy's was completely untouched.

The upcoming Monday was a holiday, so I determined I was going to D.C. on Tuesday. I didn't know what I'd do, but I was going. The next day (Saturday) was a wedding of a close friend's son. We went and tried not to be preoccupied with the catastrophe of the previous night. They are strong Believers, so I just went up to the dad and asked him to pray about the situation.

He said, "I might be able to do better than that."

He started texting away. A short while later, he gave me a name and a number. "Call her Tuesday. She'll help you get your passport expedited."

Sure enough, I received a letter from a Congressman's office via email inviting me to get an exception from the passport office.

As we were going up Tuesday morning, there was a fog hovering just high enough that when I crested the hill on I95, it made the BRAC (Military Base Realignment and Closure) building look like a mountain peeking through the clouds.

I told God, "Lord, this is our mountain. You have to move it because I can't."

I'm not sure if my faith was quite mustard-seed size that day. They asked for the letter when we arrived, and sent me in to the place for expedited passports. They told me to come back later and pick it up. Since Wednesday was a Muslim holiday and the embassy would be closed, I told them I'd come Thursday to try to pick up the passport, and then go to the embassy to get a new visa.

When I showed Thursday morning, there was a problem. They wouldn't say what. They just told me to wait.

Again, my trip was the following Monday. We were there for two to two-and-a-half hours when I finally sent an email to the Congressman's office to thank them for trying to help; that it looked like it wouldn't happen after all.

Not even a minute later, I got a response. She told me to call her office and to speak to someone there. While I got on the phone with him, the lady at the counter called me over. "I guess your emails and phone calls worked. They're bringing them down now."

Unbelievable!!

We had now about one-half hour to get to the Pakistani embassy to submit our visa applications before they closed at 12:30. That is the time they stop accepting applications. It is also lunchtime traffic in Washington, D.C.

Imagine Mission Impossible music in the background. This truly was an impossible mission. It sure seemed that way to me. But nothing's impossible with God.

We were in the office with 10 minutes to spare. This man, who had given us such a hard time last week, did not want to help us. Last week we'd seen people turned away that had been trying for six months, simply because they applied for a tourist visa. The man said, "That's fishy! Who goes to Pakistan as a tourist! Go home. No!"

Just so you know, when we turned in our damaged passports to get the new ones, we weren't able to take the new visa out, or even use the damaged passport to show as proof. When I showed him my receipt and told him what had happened, you can imagine his response.

Fortunately, I had printed out a picture of my shredded passport and showed it to him. He snatched it out of my hand and took it to a superior. He went back and forth two or three times. "Where's the picture of her passport?" he demanded, pointing at Beka.

"I thought after you saw mine you wouldn't need any more proof."

He went back for the final time. I thought we were certainly going to be rejected.

"You know you're going to have to pay for it again!"

"No problem."

We waited to show our excitement until we left the building.

We had to come back at 3:00 p.m. We paid, and got those miraculous visas.

The following Monday we made that arduous – but to us, enjoyable flight. We arrived at 3:00 a.m. Pakistan time. Even so, there were about 50 people waiting for us. Each person put a garland of flowers around our necks. After this trip, I would have expected a worldwide flower shortage. We received that kind of treatment everywhere we went.

We got to Yousaf's apartment around 5:00 a.m. They had food prepared and washed our feet. Every chance they got, someone would massage us. This is really something in their culture I've never seen anywhere else. Men that are close friends walk down the street holding hands, they massage each other, or they will put their head on a friend's lap.

They freely show love – not in a homosexual way, but truly like how families show love. It was beautiful.

Pastor Yousaf has raised up almost 470 pastors in Pakistan, so he had several large street gatherings set up. They were literally in the street. They blocked it off, covered the street with carpets and built a platform.

There was a procession at each gathering similar to in India. The difference here is we had several armed guards surrounding us – even on the platforms. These conventions would have from 300 to 400 to a couple thousand people.

The first night there were only about 350 people. When one of the leaders spoke, he tried to say there were many ways to heaven. "The Muslims say Allah, the Christians Jesus, the Jews God, the Hindus..."

You get the point. I showed Pastor the scripture God gave me for that night. John 14:6 Jesus saying, "I am the way, the truth, and the life. There is no way to the father but through me."

Yousaf read it and said, "Maybe you shouldn't."

I started praying. I knew this is what God wanted me to share. I did not want to shy away from what God called me to say. I asked Him to make a way. The man promptly approached me, excused himself and left.

I looked at Yousaf. He said, "Go for it."

Earlier that day, I was wondering if we were just going to plant seeds there, or if we would actually see a harvest of people accepting Jesus. God would soon give us the answer.

That afternoon as Yousaf showed us their women's skills center, a man asked us to enter his home and bless it and his family. This happened a lot. He explained his son was a heroin addict. We asked if we could pray for the son. The man started to cry, and gave his life to Jesus.

God answered the question if we'd see fruit or not.

That night at the first convention, only seven men came forward to receive Jesus. I thought it noteworthy because in most places, the men are harder to reach than the women. Women more easily come forward than men do to receive Christ in a setting like this where it is so public. Pakistan would prove to be the same, but this night it was only men.

Also, you have to understand the risk these men were putting themselves at by receiving Jesus publicly in a place where people will kill you for converting.

After the convention we were talking about the fact that only men came forward. The local pastor said, "You don't know the half of it. These men were the trouble makers here. They were the town drug dealers. This is a big deal!"

Wow!

Earlier in the day the drug addict came to Christ, and now the drug dealers came to Christ.

The next convention was much larger. 2,000-plus people were there. And because it was in the middle of a city setting, that number didn't include the people listening inside the buildings and from the rooftops (literally).

They brought us in a beautifully decorated, horse-drawn carriage. Hundreds of people walked down the streets with us. Beka loved it.

I remember one point I shared that has stuck with me. God gave to me that night kind of an in-the-moment inspiration that was not preplanned. I'd never quite said it like this before:

"When you buy a bottle of perfume, it's not the bottle that gives it value. It's the perfume inside the bottle. The bottle itself only carries what is of real value. It's the same with me. The only thing of value in me is the sweet aroma of Jesus. That is the only thing that gives me value. Otherwise, I am just the bottle."

That was pretty profound as I said it. It was really like I was also hearing it for the first time, even though the words came out of my mouth.

Hundreds received Jesus that night – too many to even try to count. People also asked us to pray for healing. Many people there have hepatitis C; so many women couldn't have children. I know a lot of their problems stem from the poor sanitary conditions. Huge, open canals of raw sewage run through the middle of town. The stench could knock you over, but these people are so used to it that they don't really smell it anymore. You see people sitting on the wall of the canal as if it were a local river.

Pastor Yousaf had a large team of about 20 young men that were with him constantly, doing whatever needed to be done. They all seemed proficient with cameras, video equipment, singing and playing music.

I was blown away. They threw a birthday party for Rebekah. My goodness was she spoiled by them. She cried when I told her we couldn't stay in Pakistan. She said she wanted to move there.

One day, Judy asked if they'd take her to the store. Yousaf insisted he'd make sure she had what she needed. But Judy wanted to experience shopping in Pakistan. Pastor Yousaf got very serious. "Judy, I can NEVER let you go outside. I am responsible for your safety and I can never put you in that kind of danger."

Judy said it was then that she realized how insulated, how sheltered we were from the realities of us being in Pakistan. And how much she loved the people of Pakistan, as she wanted to fully experience their culture.

They set up a convention in a completely Muslim town. Yousaf insisted that we must leave before dark because of the danger to us. I told him, "I'm along for the ride. I come and leave on your schedule."

The town was about two hours away. We went in a car they rented. All the other guys were on what I consider dirt bikes – motorcycles that are not street legal in the States. All rode two or three to one motorcycle.

Yousaf had scheduled for us to dedicate a church on the way there, and we did. In the small village, the raw sewage came out of the house right into the street. The children playing stepped over it as if it were rain water.

Everything took longer than planned. It was now getting dark, and we hadn't yet left the church.

By the time we reached the Muslim village, it was late. There was a huge *tent* set up with banners, posters, and music promoting the event. The tent was basically a wall of carpets hanging down to form the perimeter and no ceiling.

Huge crowds were everywhere we went. We waited at the local pastor's house that was directly across from where the event was set up.

So I can paint you a picture of this – ALL the pastors' houses were the same – it was really just a bedroom. Everyone gathered together either on the floor, or whatever little furniture they had. Most sat on the bed. This was common everywhere we went. The bedroom is where all activity took place.

I stepped outside to see all the commotion, and Pastor had a couple of guys rush me back inside. "You cannot stand outside like that. It is too dangerous!"

I felt like we were on house arrest, and it didn't make sense to me since we were going to be on that stage in a few minutes. But they know their culture best.

When we walked across to the event, they had separate entrances for the men and for the women. They had the typical armed security that the other places had, but also several uniformed police there to protect us. There were easily 1,500 people there, and many more outside the tent. The sound system was powerful so that everyone in that town would hear my message.

As happened everywhere else, the mayor came and made a few comments (basically endorsing the event) and then left. Yousaf said, "Don't worry; he will hear you in his bedroom."

God gave me the most powerful salvation message I'd ever given anywhere that night.

"If you are hearing my voice you are without excuse. You can no longer say I didn't know. And it doesn't matter what you believe, or why you believed it. Every one of us will one day face our creator regardless if you think so or not.

"And what are you going to say? You can't blame it on your family. You can't say I was told this or I was told that!

"God will be speaking to you and to you alone. There are no do-overs on this!

"He will say, 'I sent to you my Son, my prophets, and my messengers. And still you do not believe.'

"And now you've heard me. What more proof do you need? I couldn't save myself. The doctors couldn't save me. God saved me. What more proof do you need? What excuse can you now give to Him?"

Over half of that gathering came up to receive Jesus that night. I asked Yousaf, "Do they realize I did an altar call?"

He said, "Exactly. They are all coming to receive Christ."

I went down and started praying for each one when I was pulled back up to the platform. Yousaf said that the people outside the tent want to hear me pray for their salvation also.

It was the same in India. Not everyone had the courage to enter the tent because of the fear of the backlash they'd receive. Most of them were Muslim, and they were scared of the reaction of their relatives and friends. Nonetheless, they felt the power, and answered the call.

Praise God!

When I finished, I stepped down. There was an imam or mullah waiting for me. He asked me to pray for him. "In the name of Jesus..."

I was thrilled. Even after that, this man stayed by me – all the way to the car and until we left. One of the uniformed policemen, who aren't permitted to touch you, took me by the hand. He interlocked his fingers with mine as he walked me to the car. This is a very intimate type of expression of love. I've never held hands like that with any man, but he was just showing his love for me. Really interesting. Yousaf told me that was a big deal because he was a Muslim man, and my story must have resonated with him.

We also visited a brick colony. The Christians, whether born-again, or just born into a Christian household, are treated as less than human. I asked, "How can anyone know?"

They said, "By the name."

So even if you didn't believe, but you had the name John, you were treated as poorly as all the other Christians. Many are living and working at brick kilns. These are almost like forced labor camps. They are *free*, but not really. They don't get paid enough to pay the basic living expenses, so they get into debt, and are literally in servitude to their debtors.

As it says in the Bible, "Borrowers are slaves to the lenders."

And there, they really are. You can give your daughter to them as a wife and they will forgive your debt. Otherwise, you will be their slave and so will your children. This can go for generations. Pastor Yousaf has bought many people their freedom by paying their family's debt.

We have also started schools for the children to try to break the cycle their families have been in for decades.

I used the bathroom at this colony, and they took me to the owner's house. He at least had a hole in the floor. Judy used the bathroom at one of the villagers' homes. It had no hole – you just went on the floor and they washed it into the street.

It was there that Beka was baptized along with 20 or so villagers. The Christian well was broken, so they asked to use a

Muslim man's well. The algae on the bottom of the basin we stood in was thick and slippery. This was the water they used for everything, including drinking. No wonder so many are sick.

The final day, they scheduled an early conference. It was at 3:00 p.m., and we needed to be at the airport about two hours later. Since it was at the Christian colony, I didn't expect many to come forward to receive Jesus, but I did an alter call anyway.

Again, half the group came forward. I was perplexed. Yousaf told me there were many that came from outside the village, and many in the village had only been Christian by title – not in their heart. It was in their heart after that day.

Pastor Yousaf's ministry is one I love to support financially. There aren't any tax credits for supporting his ministry because it has no base in the U.S, but that's not why I support ministries anyway. I have supported large multimillion-dollar ministries for years, but they have hundreds of thousands of donors.

God really touched my heart to help ministries like these:

Yousaf in Pakistan, Herrera in Cuba, and Rajan in India.

They are struggling and changing lives in oppression most will never understand. They are doing this largely on their own. I've seen each of their ministries personally in action. I wish there was more I could do to help them continue their work.

The saddest thing is that they spend so much money and time coming to raise funds for their ministries here in the U.S. I host these pastors when they come, and try to help get them into different local churches to share. So often – and it really makes me sad – churches don't *have time* for them, or worse, meet with them and tell them they'll help them, but never do.

If they only knew what I knew. If they only saw what I have seen, it would be impossible for them to continue to maintain their ambivalence.

The vision the Holy Spirit gave Tim has definitely come true.

PS – Yousaf told me that in Pakistan if someone is burned on 40% of their body, their family will instruct the doctor to euthanize them. To just "Give them the needle."

Soul Warrior

The German writer and statesman Goethe said, "If you treat a man as they are, you make them worse. If you treat them how they ought to be, you help them become that."

Curtis reminds me of what Goethe said. I will tell you about Curtis later.

I have talked about several of the different countries I've been able to share in, but some of the most memorable times I've shared have been not the large crowds but the one-on-ones. I share whether in the grocery line with the clerk, riding in an elevator or with my servers while at restaurants. Almost every time I eat at a sit-down restaurant, I ask the server what I can pray for them about as I'm getting ready to pray for my meal.

I've received every response you could imagine – from no thanks, to people weeping at our table as we prayed with them. One young man asked us to pray for a serious situation that he couldn't disclose to us. Of course, I gave him a card with a link to the YouTube video about my testimony. Weeks later, I received an email from him. He thanked me for the prayer and the tip. The response I sent was simple, but yet profound. "God is good, even if circumstances are not."

And as God often does, He used the words coming out of my mouth (or more accurately, out of my typing fingers) to minister to me.

It's cool when you are able to see things come full circle. When you finally see all the pieces of the puzzle fall into place – getting to see the picture God has been painting all along. The seemingly disjointed events being knit together to show a master plan unfolding before your eyes – the hand of the King in action.

Reactions to witnessing range from complete ambivalence to coming completely undone. Often people do a double-take when the words actually sink in, because it really is unbelievable to imagine that happening to someone. I can share the nuts and bolts of it in about 20 seconds. That allows me to get a card in their hand so they can watch the video later. In most cases it encourages people.

Here's the URL that is on the card my wife prepared for me to hand out to people:

https://www.youtube.com/watch?v=4cGV6ASLFK0&feature=youtu.be

I remember walking my father through the sinner's prayer. Dad was the first one I witnessed to. And the first to say, "Yes" to Jesus; a friend since I was a teenager who was a devout atheist and now calls Jesus Lord; and the very first homeless man that gave his life to Jesus after hearing my story. What I really remember most is the truly repentant weeping. Seeing that (as well as baptisms) can usually bring tears to my eyes, and most definitely bring joy to my heart.

Now the lead-in to how I met Curtis. You will see how these seemingly unrelated events, tied together, are unleashing another miraculous work. Another life being changed.

To God be the glory!

My daughter Beka went to a Christian academy for pre-k 3, and pre-k 4. At the end of the second year, the teacher recommended holding her back. She just didn't think Beka was ready. Since her birthday is in September, it didn't seem to be that big of a deal. At the end of the second go-round of pre-k 4, her teacher again recommended she be held back.

"I don't think so."

My wife suggested we get her eyes checked as one of her older children had a similar issue. She was tested, and Judy was right. Beka wasn't able to focus binocularly. Almost like she was seeing everything through a prism. Could you imagine how hard it would be to learn letters and numbers like that?

We went through over a year of therapy with the doctor, and homeschooled her for kindergarten. We taught her how to read, and taught her three-digit addition and subtraction, money counting, and beginning fractions.

She excelled being homeschooled. The following year, she was so far advanced that I not only thought that she was ready to go to school again, I thought she might skip first grade and be put into second.

Beka wanted us to continue homeschooling. She loved being at home with us.

But we went to the same school she had gone to before hoping to ease the transition. To me there wasn't even a question of where she'd go.

God was about to show me I was wrong.

On the day of the assessment, I guess Beka froze up. They said they couldn't get enough from her to determine if she could even enter kindergarten. She was not allowed to go to that school unless I brought a note from a doctor to let them know "what's wrong with her."

I said, "I think this conversation has run its course." And I stormed out.

To say I was upset would be an understatement. God slammed that door in my face, probably because I was too hard-headed to ask where He wanted her to go.

He was about to open another door.

We went to two other academies – not all private schools are Christian.

Judy asked, "Are we going to sacrifice her spiritual well-being for the lure of the superior education that was painted for us?"

At both academies they thought that she not only was ready for first grade, but recognized that she was advanced and they could speed up the pace for her to keep her ahead.

My best friend Tim called me in the middle of all this. "What you doing?"

"Looking at schools for Beka."

Tim told me about a school I'd never heard of, but sounded like it was worth checking out'

When we called, they only had one slot left. We went right away to check it out. We connected immediately with the owners of the school, Scott and Stacie. They were down-to-earth, and completely sold out for Jesus.

The other thing that astounded me was that their son had a similar vision issue like Beka did, and used the same doctor we did. Stacie taught him, and she was to be the teacher that would teach Beka's class.

On top of all this amazingness, they had farm animals: a goat, chickens. Rabbits in the classroom.

Beka would be right at home. It couldn't be a better situation. They also started a ministry for youth where they had free food and music once a month. I mentioned that I played bass, and they said, "That's the only thing we don't have, a bass player."

I thought *How cool is that?*

As we did the tour, we also met the woman that would be Stacie's classroom assistant. That was her first day working there. Her name was Tari. Stacie told me God told Tari to take the job with the academy and how lucky she felt to have her.

As I often do, I handed Tari my card and gave a thumbnail description of the story. She read my name. "Peter Dechat? You are Peter Dechat? Pete Dechat?"

She was stunned.

"I'm not famous, ok?"

Her reaction baffled me. She didn't tell me right away, but I later found out from Stacie that five days earlier she was praying with a mutual friend. In the middle of praying, this friend blurted out, "Do you know Pete Dechat?"

When Tari said, "No" the friend said, "Too bad. You really need to meet him."

Now I understood her reaction.

By the end of the week, she had invited me to share my testimony at a homeless ministry. So I did. I now play with Tari on the house worship team for the once-a-month conferences.

One day Tari told me the pastors of the homeless ministry were going on vacation for a week. That they had been ministering to one homeless man in particular, and were worried about him for that time they'd be gone. They asked Tari to ask me if I could reach out to him that week. So I got his name and number:

Curtis.

This is a name you will want to remember. This man lost his wife and three young sons in a house fire in 2008. I had no idea what was about to unfold. I sent him a text letting him know that the pastors from the ministry asked me to call him. He called back right away. Judy was sitting next to me as I took his call. I had it on speaker phone, and the expletives started flying. Judy asked me to mute the phone and she said, "I guess we reached a new level of ministry."

He was angry, hated everyone and everything. He said he was drinking every day and just couldn't get out of 2008. I talked with him three times that day. I was blown away by the things he was telling me. His story is so unbelievable, all the things he's been through.

I told him, "I've often wondered why God saved me in that accident. It may have been just so I can meet you. The call God has for your life may be greater than mine. You are so important spiritually that the demons have been trying to crush your life since before you were even born."

I am one of a very small number of people who could understand what he's been through, just as he is one of a very small number of people who could understand what I've been through. Yes, the circumstances are different, but I can understand his pain and he can understand mine.

I spoke to him every day, multiple times a day. He has shared things with me that he's shared with no one else. I encouraged him, prayed with him, and for him. Slowly, his language changed. He started coming to church. He stopped drinking. He's not out of the woods yet, but he's in the Bible every day. The enemy is still scratching and clawing at him, trying to pull him back in. His is a story still being written, but his is a name you will want to remember. I love this man, and believe God is going to raise him up to save many lives through the testimony still being woven together.

One night my good friend Mike Zello, the director of Teen Challenge here in central Virginia, allowed me to go share my testimony. I brought Curtis with me and they allowed him to share his story too. That was the first place he shared his story with anyone. I am so proud of him and all the changes that he's made in his life. He continues to strive to better himself and I can see Jesus in him more and more with every step he takes.

I can't wait for this story to be written:

"Hello, my name is Curtis..."

Postscript

Even when I lay in the hospital, I knew I would eventually write this book. I would even get flashes of scenes, as if I were watching a movie. Whatever the format, I knew this story had to get out.

I remember being in church at River of Life, and a friend came up to me somewhat unsure. He said, "I don't know what this means, but God said to start writing."

He looked very uncomfortable as he said it.

"I've never come up to anyone like this before, but that's what He wants me to tell you – start writing."

I knew what it meant. God had to use someone else to tell me because I was obviously ignoring Him.

"I will," I said.

I actually hired a ghostwriter to help me, but he got very ill. Long story short: five years later there was still no book.

In that time I had more people tell I me I should write a book than I can count. And I can count pretty high, at least to 27. Ok that was a joke. I can actually count to 28. Seriously, there have been hundreds.

Anyway, I finally went back to him. "I understand you're sick, but God told ME to write this book. I won't be able to stand before Him and say, 'But the writer was sick.' I will have to answer for why I didn't get it done. I can't blame anyone else."

I just wanted the notes back so I could get started.

Around the same time, a very good friend of mine, Tim Shields, who runs the Christian Media Alliance, was telling me about their annual conference in Dallas. Tim's son was my wife's son's best friend. I've known him for many years. He'd told me what he did for a living, but I never really got it.

A month or two before he mentioned this conference, I asked him to explain what he did again. He did.

I proceeded. "I don't know why I haven't asked you about this, but I feel God wants me to make a movie or write a book about my testimony.

Tim is always super polite, and I felt like he was trying to protect my feelings a bit.

"Well, it would have to be really compelling. Most people just aren't interested."

I had to stop. "Wait . . . how many years have I known you? You don't know my testimony?"

"I know a little."

I sent him the YouTube link with the video. Not more than five minutes later he sent a response:

"Now that's compelling!"

Fast forward to this time when he brought up the conference. I've supported his ministry for years, but never truly understood it. I just knew he was a Godly man doing God's work. This time, however, he said, "We have three keynote speakers. If you can sponsor one of them I can show your testimony video and give you a minute to talk about it."

I jumped at that. I thought *God, I don't know what you're cooking here, but I don't want to let this opportunity pass by.*

Anne Graham Lotz was the keynote speaker I sponsored. I didn't even know who she was.

Coincidentally, Tim also invited our church's worship leader to bring a team down. I got to play there as well. It was an amazing time, and I got to meet a lot of people in Christian media.

When we were leaving, we were three hours early to the airport. We flew out of the smaller of the two Dallas airports. We got through security quickly. With so much time to kill, Judy and I decided to find a nice sit-down restaurant. We checked out all of them before deciding on one. As our food arrived, and we started eating, Judy leaned across the table. "Hey, I think they were at the conference," pointing to the couple that was just seated right next to us. "They won one of the awards. I recognize her shirt."

They were literally close enough to eat off of our plates.

Of all the restaurants in the airport they chose this one. Of all the seats in this restaurant, they were seated right next to us. God is good.

Being the shy one I am, I said, "Hey! I know you. You were at the conference."

Because I played on the worship team and shared about my testimony they recognized us as well.

We really hit it off with them. It was Wes and Amanda Llewellyn. They are producers/directors.

In the middle of the conversation, Wes stopped. "I don't usually say things like this, but God's not TELLING me you need to write a book. He's SCREAMING it in my ear!"

I felt totally convicted, and explained how I tried – really just sounded like a bunch of excuses.

They said they knew a great ghostwriter, Jim Dobkins, but he was busy on a project. They seemed really excited for me. We kept in touch after this.

Two or three weeks after the conference, Amanda texted me. "The writer finished his project."

I wasted no time. I texted him right away, but got no response. Life got busy, and I didn't think about it for about two weeks. I thought maybe he wasn't interested in writing my story. Out of the blue, I decided I'd call. What a noble concept. Try to actually speak to someone. Found out Jim does not do texting.

The rest is history.

Why I hand out my card

I share my testimony all the time. Whether with a waitress, grocery clerk, wherever. When the tube was in my throat I couldn't speak at all. Since God gave me my voice back I'm going to use it.

I remember being invited by Theresa Mills from WPER radio in Virginia to share my testimony at one of their annual dinners. She and I had become good friends over the years of me supporting their ministry. They had comedian Marty Simpson as the entertainment for the evening and I shared right before him.

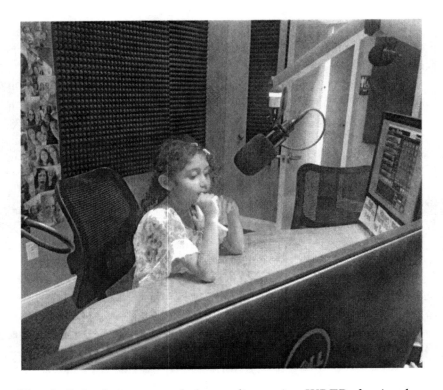

Here's Beka being recorded at radio station WPER sharing her version of my testimony.

After I spoke, which was only a few minutes, he was brought on. His opening was, "As comedians we share with each other the toughest act we had to follow. I just texted everyone – that this was it."

He went on with his act and he was hilarious.

Afterwards I met him by the exit. He asked me for a card.

"I'm not important enough to have a card," I said.

"I can understand," he said seriously. "I mean, cards can run $29. I can see why you don't have them."

Cracked me up.

Anyway, Judy, the brains of our operation, made cards for me for my birthday to make sharing my testimony easier. She asked how many I wanted. I go by the belief that if a little is good, a lot is better. We ordered 10,000 of them. As crazy as that sounds, I may already be half-way through them after one year.

Theresa invited me to another WPER event which was a breakfast. The lead singer for Tenth Avenue North, Mike Donehey, was going to be there. I didn't even know who he was, but went anyway. Over the next couple of months I would see him at other events. At one of them for the Choices Women's Center annual gala dinner in Fredericksburg, there he was AGAIN!

When leaving the event, I said to Judy kind of in passing, "I think I'm supposed to meet him." I didn't want to say, "God told me," because it could've been the food, but it just seemed too coincidental to me.

Two days later, Theresa asked if I wanted to go to a Tenth Avenue North concert she had tickets to. Judy was surprised at how quickly I jumped at it. When she asked what that was all about, I reminded her of the Choices gala the week before. She immediately got it.

We were there for the Q&A before the concert, and I actually did get to introduce myself to him before the concert. He was already late, and talking to people he knew out front. As shy as I am, I waited right next to him to introduce myself. With only 10 seconds to make my not-so-good first impression, I handed him my card and said, "I don't know why, but I think I'm supposed to meet you." I'm sure His one word synopsis that meeting would probably be ". . . creepy."

However short and awkward that meeting was, I did learn some powerful lessons from him. I preface this by saying that he, nor the group Tenth Avenue North, need my endorsement. They don't even know I exist. They are wildly popular, and I give God praise and thanks that they are. As a musician, of course, I love their talent and professionalism of their group. But my takeaway was more like, "Oh, and they play music too."

The messages before, during, and after the music were so powerful, relevant and relatable, it's no wonder God has given them this platform. God is glorified every chance they get.

The other thing, which is more for me personally, was that this man, though famous, and incredibly pressed for time, was 100% present while talking with everyone I saw him interact with, including me. I needed to see this because I have the attention span of a two-year-old. If I'm ever talking with you and you notice me distracted, or I start chasing a squirrel around the backyard, please give me grace. I need it.

Nothing says love like giving your time, and your focused attention. The Bible says to give honor where honor is due, and Mike deserves it. Whereas I hope he doesn't remember that chance meeting, I will never forget it.

More about the author

Grow your own

We finished and moved into our forever house in August 2013. One of my goals was to be able to be self-sufficient if it was ever a necessity.

Part of that desire to be self-sufficient was to also grow a percentage of what we eat. The more I've learned about the mass production of the food in the grocery stores, even organic, the more I wanted to grow my own.

God really had a good plan:

Eat foods in season, from your surroundings. I would love to see more people use the local butcher, local bread maker, and local cheese maker. It would be leaps and bounds better for our health as a society than the mass food production that comes from who knows where, and is sprayed with who knows what.

When I later went to Cuba, I was shocked at the level of obesity. It wasn't because of the abundance of food, but the abundance of BAD food.

The same problem is rampant in this country, especially for the poor. How is it possible to sell a cheeseburger for less than a stalk of broccoli? The cheeseburger is more filling, the broccoli healthier; but if you have a hungry child and no money, you choose what fills their belly more.

A lot of the chemicals, which can now be sprayed directly on many crops, have been shown to kill our good-gut bacteria in the same way it kills weeds.

The good-gut bacteria produce many of the chemicals that keep us emotionally balanced. It's no wonder depression and anxiety are on the rise.

No one is going to care as much for your wellbeing, and your family's wellbeing, as you will. I wanted to take back control of what we were consuming.

I don't grow as much of our food as I'd like, but I'm learning. I've been getting milk from my goats for two years, but I'm the only one drinking it. I have made a great deal of cheese from it. We get eggs from the chickens. We started our first beehive, so next year we should get some honey. I make an amazing bread where I actually mill the flour from sprouted grains.

We get hundreds of pounds of strawberries and blackberries, but because we do everything organic, and never have the time to pick them all, our chickens get about half of them because they go bad before they get picked. This year I got a lot of tomatoes and Asian eggplants. One of my new favorite dishes to make is with those two ingredients along with fresh oregano. Our watermelons also did well this year. Do I want more? Of course.

Next year I expect to be better because I'm realizing some of my mistakes. I also need to succession plant so that we can enjoy a more spread-out harvesting period.

We also enjoy potatoes, apples, persimmons, and a few other fruits, but not enough to write home about. We even got a pineapple and some limes from the tropical plants that need to be taken in every year.

Last year, I taught the Dave Ramsey Financial Peace University. Part of our new budgeting was to cut our eating out in half. This has been so great. The financial benefits are obvious: tax is roughly 2-3% for food in the grocery store where I live, and 12% for food at restaurants. No restaurant can cook a meal for the same price you can cook a meal. Also, you know what you're eating, especially if you grow it. You know that the average restaurant is watching food costs and profits closer than the health risks their food might cause you.

But on top of all that, I've realized that I really like to cook. I was truly blessed to have a friend that was a trained chef. He started a business that I wanted to support, so we hired him to cook for us often. I watched what he was doing and learned some of his techniques.

In conclusion, there is one more thing I'm really excited to tell you about.

Judy is writing her story, which is every bit as powerful as my testimony. Watch for it:

Romanced By The King

And if you have not yet seen my YouTube testimony video, please watch it right now. I owe special thanks to Tawaan Brown from Beyond Creativity for making this video; also, the video about our visit to Pakistan.

https://www.youtube.com/watch?v=4cGV6ASLFK0&feature=youtu.be

Do you have questions for Pete?
Want to know when he might be speaking near you?
When and where he will be next signing books?
Or do you want to schedule him for a speaking engagement?
You can follow Pete at his special web site for all of these details and more:

www.ThroughTheFire.net

And if you really love this book, please let the world know by writing a review of the print and ebook editions on Pete's web site, and at other Internet venues where good reviews can increase a book's success.

CPSIA information can be obtained
at www.ICGtesting.com
Printed in the USA
FFOW01n1950070418
46152757-47331FF